The Nd-YAG Laser in Ophthalmology

Principles and Clinical Applications of Photodisruption

ROGER F. STEINERT, M.D.

CARMEN A. PULIAFITO, M.D.

Department of Ophthalmology, Massachusetts Eye and Ear
Infirmary, Harvard Medical School, Boston, Massachusetts;
Regional Laser Center, George R. Harrison Spectroscopy
Laboratory, Massachusetts Institute of Technology,
Cambridge, Massachusetts

1985

W. B. SAUNDERS COMPANY

Philadelphia/London/Toronto/Mexico City/Rio de Janeiro/Sydney/Tokyo

W. B. Saunders Company: West Washington Square
Philadelphia, PA   19105

1 St. Anne's Road
Eastbourne, East Sussex BN21 3UN, England

1 Goldthorne Avenue
Toronto, Ontario M8Z 5T9, Canada

Apartado 26370—Cedro 512
Mexico 4, D.F., Mexico

Rua Coronel Cabrita, 8
Sao Cristovao Caixa Postal 21176
Rio de Janeiro, Brazil

9 Waltham Street
Artarmon, N.S.W. 2064, Australia

Ichibancho, Central Bldg., 22-1 Ichibancho
Chiyoda-Ku, Tokyo 102, Japan

Library of Congress Cataloging in Publication Data

Steinert, Roger F.

The Nd-YAG laser in ophthalmology.

1. Eye—Surgery.   2. Lasers in surgery.   3. Neodymium-
yttrium aluminum garnet lasers.   I. Puliafito, Carmen A.,
1951– .   II. Title. [DNLM: 1. Eye Diseases—surgery.
2. Lasers—therapeutic use. WW 168 S822n]

RE80.S66 1985   617.7'1   84–14046

ISBN 0–7216–1320–9

THE Nd-YAG LASER IN OPHTHALMOLOGY:
Principles and Clinical Applications of Photodisruption   ISBN   0-7216-1320-9

Last digit is the print number: 9   8   7   6   5   4   3   2   1

*Dedicated to
our families*

ACKNOWLEDGMENTS

The pioneer work of Drs. Danielle Aron-Rosa and Franz Fankhauser and their colleagues brought photodisruption with the Nd-YAG laser into safe and effective clinical therapeutics. For this all ophthalmologists are in their debt. Dr. Aron-Rosa has welcomed and encouraged our work from the outset, and we thank her for her support.

This book would not have been possible without the help of many individuals. We owe a particular debt of gratitude to many members of the scientific communities at the Massachusetts Institute of Technology and Harvard University, who welcomed us into their laboratories and generously made available their time and resources. Our first experimental studies in short-pulsed laser research were performed at the Regional Laser Center and the George R. Harrison Laboratory of Spectroscopy at MIT. Special thanks must go to Dr. Michael S. Feld, Director of the Regional Laser Center, and Drs. Carter Kittrell and Ramachandra Dasari. Drs. James G. Fujimoto and Erich P. Ippen of the MIT Department of Electrical Engineering provided early technical support as well as ideas and have become valued collaborators. Dr. Kevin Peters of the Harvard Chemistry Department provided ready access to his scientific mode-locked laser system.

At the Massachusetts Eye and Ear Infirmary, where all of our clinical work has been done, Drs. David L. Epstein and Evangelos S. Gragoudas have provided invaluable support of many kinds. Dr. Claudia U. Richter has been instrumental in organizing clinical research in the laser center. Dr. Daniel M. Albert and Mr. Joseph L. Craft made our first morphologic studies possible. Drs. S. Arthur Boruchoff and Charles D. J. Regan provided encouragement and wisdom. Dr. Claes H. Dohlman, our Chief and Department Chairman, has supported our efforts both materially and emotionally. Dr. Ephraim Friedman, Infirmary President, has been an enthusiastic supporter of the laser research program from the outset. Two talented residents, Drs. Paul J. Wasson and Mark A. Latina, were early and important collaborators. Catherine Adler, our research assistant, has worked tirelessly in organizing the laser research laboratory.

Invaluable support has been provided by Dr. William J. Link, Dr. Stephen M. Fry, Paul R. Goth, and Dr. Edward G. Malk. We are grateful for their help.

Dr. R. Rox Anderson and Dr. John A. Parrish of the Massachusetts General Hospital have shared with us their insights into photobiology. Drs. Richard H. Keates, Stephen L. Trokel, and Manus Kraff provided advice, encouragement, and support on many occasions.

Drs. Thomas Hanscom, Douglas Gaasterland, Stephen Johnson, Richard

Kratz, John Hunkeler, Paul Woodward, Thomas Richardson, and David Epstein kindly made available case material and photographs for this book. Laurel Cook skillfully prepared the line drawings and interpreted clinical concepts in her beautiful artwork. Linda Mikula artfully drafted the charts. Alan Ball provided excellent administrative and secretarial support, without which the book would not have been possible.

Critical to the success of this venture and the laser research laboratory has been the continuing support of the Donaldson Trust.

To the patients who participated in the clinical studies reported in this book we owe a special debt. In many ways, these patients were co-investigators whose enthusiasm and hope has helped us to carry forward our inquiries.

Finally, we acknowledge our parents, who provided the foundation, our wives, Dr. Marilyn Steinert and Dr. Janet Pine, who gave daily encouragement, advice, and support, and our children, who inspire us with curiosity and enthusiasm.

ROGER F. STEINERT, M.D.

CARMEN A. PULIAFITO, M.D.

PREFACE

Photodisruption is the mechanical alteration of an object by an extremely powerful ionizing electromagnetic field associated with radiation in the portion of the electromagnetic spectrum defined as "light" (ultraviolet, visible, and infrared). In ophthalmology, the Q-switched and mode-locked neodymium-yttrium-aluminum-garnet (Nd-YAG) lasers are clinical photodisruptors. By emitting light pulses lasting billionths to trillionths of a second, focused to a spot the size of a white blood cell, these lasers create such a strong electromagnetic field that electrons are torn from their atoms, and a strong localized pressure wave results. This process is known as optical breakdown.

This book is intended for the ophthalmologist who wishes to understand photodisruption and apply it therapeutically to the eye. No prior knowledge of lasers, physics, or photobiology is assumed.

Section I explores the principles of photobiology and lasers in general and of photodisruption in particular. After the history of phototherapy of ocular disease and the development of photodisruption are reviewed, the special properties of laser light are introduced. Physics and mathematics are restricted to pertinent major concepts. Optical breakdown, plasma formation, and photodisruption are explained, and a detailed discussion of laser-tissue interaction follows. These chapters are intended as a foundation for understanding not only current laser technology but future developments as well. Section I concludes with a chapter on Nd-YAG lasers and ophthalmic delivery systems, both to explain engineering goals and constraints and to serve as a buyer's and user's guide to current and future commercial lasers.

Section II is devoted to clinical applications of Q-switched and mode-locked ophthalmic Nd-YAG lasers. Section II may be used independently of Section I. Section II begins with a review of the important principles of optical breakdown in clinical applications. Liberal reference is made to the relevant areas in Section I that support and explain the principles of critical focus. Each chapter on applications then reviews the current literature in that area, presents illustrative cases with discussion of indications and complications, and concludes with a summary of patient preparation, operative technique, and postoperative care.

This book should serve as a coherent teaching text and as a reference source. While we have attempted to be comprehensive and objective in our treatment of the subject, this work must also reflect our personal experiences and viewpoints. We apologize for any inaccuracies that result. Your comments, criticisms, and suggestions are encouraged.

ROGER F. STEINERT, M.D.

CARMEN A. PULIAFITO, M.D.

CONTENTS

13
POSTERIOR SEGMENT APPLICATIONS 134

APPENDIX 138

PLATE I

A Four millimeter posterior capsulotomy behind a posterior chamber intraocular lens.

B Coreoplasty to restore the optical axis to the central cornea. The pupil was drawn upward to the left after wound leak following intracapsular cataract extraction and was covered by the eyelid in its normal position. Arrowheads indicate the pupillary border before sphincterotomy.

C Aphakic malignant glaucoma with apposition of inferior iris to edematous cornea.

D Depth is restored to the anterior chamber immediately after Nd-YAG laser pulses have opened the anterior hyaloid face. Arrows show separation of iris and cornea, in comparison with IC.

E Pupillary block glaucoma with loss of anterior chamber one day after intracapsular cataract extraction with anterior chamber intraocular lens implant. Hemorrhage covers the implant optic, and the iris is in apposition to the superior cornea, except where the edge of the optic creates a small aqueous lacuna (*arrow*).

F Postlaser photograph of patient in IE. Immediately after Nd-YAG laser iridectomy, the chamber begins to form, with aqueous space between the superior iris and the hemorrhage-covered optic (*arrows*).

G Gonioscopy shows the iris drawn upward into the angle in a tentlike formation as a result of vitreous incarceration in the wound. The arrow indicates the iris deformation and the arrowhead the adjacent peripheral iridectomy. Figure 10–4*A* shows the slit lamp appearance of this eye.

H Appearance of angle shown in IG after laser vitreolysis. The pigmented trabecular meshwork is now visible (*arrow*) adjacent to the peripheral iridectomy (*arrowhead*). Figure 10–4C shows the slit lamp appearance of the same eye at this stage of the procedure.

PLATE I

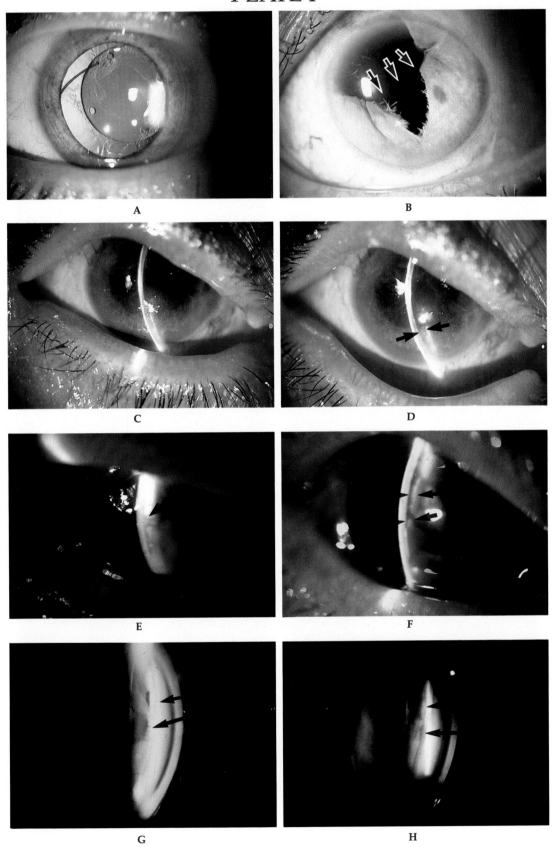

PLATE II

A   A strand of vitreous humor to the wound is present in association with cystoid macular edema. A fine wisp of vitreous passes from the pupil (*arrowhead*) across the peripheral iridectomy to the wound (*arrow*). Figure 10–5A shows the slit lamp appearance of this pupil.

B   After laser vitreolysis, the strand seen in IIA is gone. A fine hemorrhage can be seen at the edge of the peripheral iridectomy (*arrow*) and is caused by the pressure wave emanating from the zone of optical breakdown anterior to the iridectomy.

C   A retained fragment of anterior capsule after extracapsular cataract extraction is in contact with the corneal endothelium. Localized stromal thickening can be seen in the slit beam (*arrow*).

D   After laser disruption of the capsule shown in IIC, the corneal edema has resolved. A small fragment of capsule remains adherent to the endothelium (*arrow*).

E   Preoperative laser anterior capsulotomy. Vacuoles have been created centrally by laser shots in the anterior cortex behind the anterior capsule. A series of closely spaced shots has formed a nearly complete circular anterior capsulotomy in the mid-periphery. (Courtesy of Paul M. Woodward.)

F   Appearance of the lens in IIE the next day, 18 hours after anterior capsulotomy. The cortex has become opaque owing to hydration through the anterior capsule defects. (Courtesy of Paul M. Woodward.)

G   Preoperative photograph of the fundus. This patient had a history of long-term uveitis in this eye, with opacification of the posterior hyaloid membrane and a nasal traction detachment. (Courtesy of Thomas A. Hanscom.)

H   Postoperative photograph of the fundus. After two treatments employing 650 pulses with energies up to 8 mJ, the membrane was successfully cut (*arrows*). (Courtesy of Thomas A. Hanscom.)

PLATE II

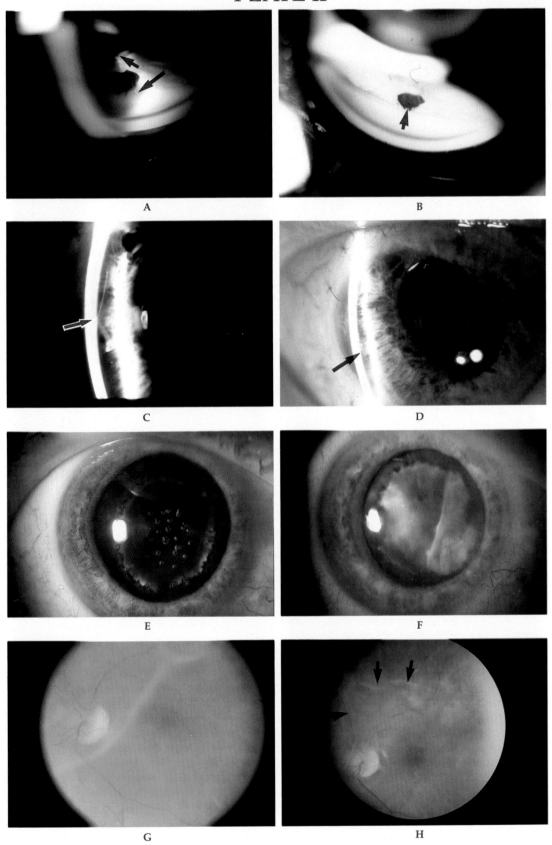

The Nd-YAG Laser in Ophthalmology

Principles and Clinical Applications
of Photodisruption

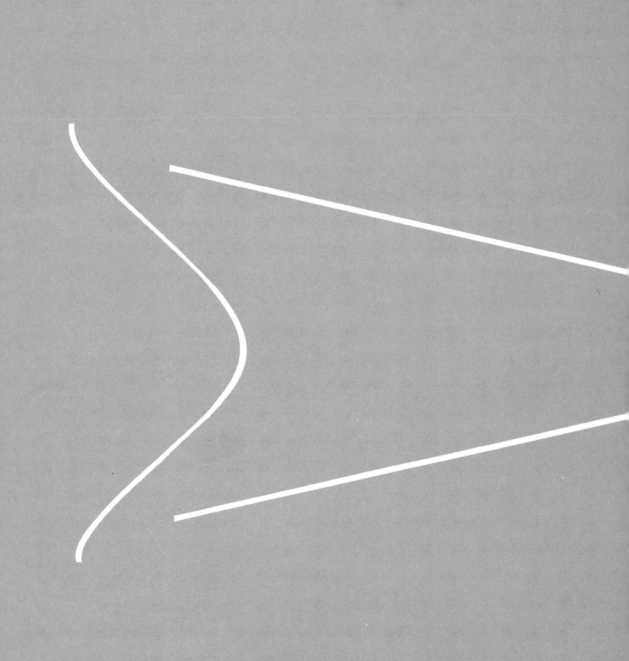

SECTION I

PRINCIPLES

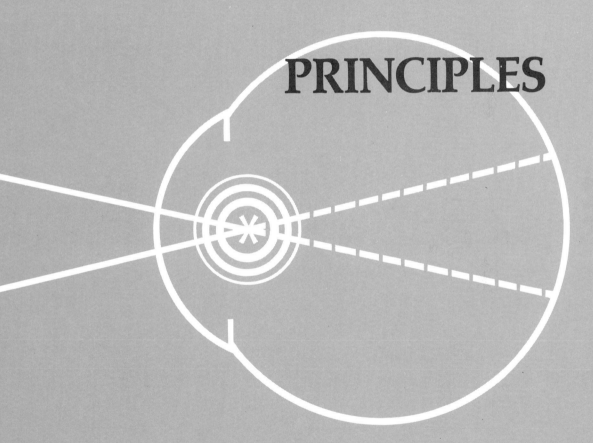

1
HISTORICAL
CONSIDERATIONS

The recognition that the radiant energy of the sun could damage the human eye was a first step in the development of ocular phototherapy. Solar retinitis (eclipse blindness) was recognized by the ancients. This quotation from Plato's *Phaidon* is often cited: " 'When I had given up inquiring into real evidence,' Socrates proceeded, 'I thought that I must take care that I did not suffer as people who look at the sun during eclipse. For they are apt to lose their eyesight unless they look at the sun's reflection in water or some such medium. That danger occurred to me. I was afraid that my soul might be completely blinded if I looked at things with my eyes and tried to grasp them with my senses.' "[1]

Bonetus, an ophthalmologist practicing in Geneva in the seventeenth century, is credited with being the first to describe the occurrence of a scotoma after sun gazing.[2] Czerny (1867) and Deutschmann (1882) focused sunlight on the retinas of rabbits by means of a concave mirror and convex lens and noted the appearance of grayish burns, which eventually produced hyperpigmented scars.[3, 4] Verhoeff, Bell, and Walker's monumental 1916 monograph *Pathologic Effects of Radiant Energy on the Eye* was an important contribution to the developing field of photobiology.[5]

The modern history of photocoagulation began with the work of Gerd Meyer-Schwickerath, a young ophthalmologist at the University of Hamburg. He demonstrated that focused radiant energy could be used to create chorioretinal lesions of clinical value. His interest was aroused by personal observation of several patients who had sustained macular damage during the solar eclipse of the sun on July 10, 1945. One of the patients had a small pigmented macular scar that resembled the scar resulting from diathermy. Meyer-Schwickerath's struggle to identify a suitable light source and to develop a workable delivery system was not easy. Light from high-voltage incandescent lamps, high-pressure mercury lamps, and carbon arcs was considered. The first source to be tried clinically in photocoagulation in the human eye was the carbon arc. Unfortunately, the intensities of radiation required to produce a lesion in the human eye were greater than those required for the rabbit eye and could not be attained with the carbon arc then available.

At this point, Meyer-Schwickerath turned his attention once again to the sun. He developed a photocoagulator that used the sun as its light source. This

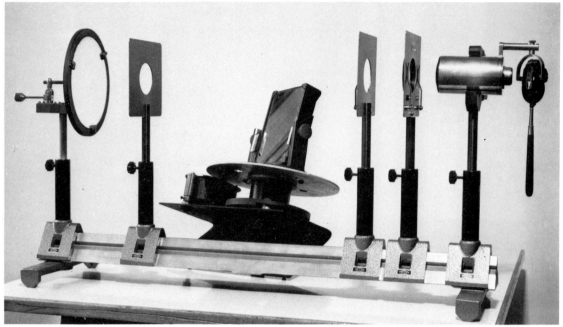

FIGURE 1–1   Sunlight photocoagulator. On the right, the Galilean telescope with a direct ophthalmoscope on a universal joint. On the left, a mirror and heliostat. (Courtesy of Gerd Meyer-Schwickerath)

instrument, illustrated in Figure 1–1, consisted of a Galilean telescope with a mirror that had a central aperture and was suspended on a universal joint in front of the ocular. This instrument produced Meyer-Schwickerath's first clinical successes. However, the frequent occurrence of cloudy days in Northern Europe made the sunlight photocoagulator impractical. Meyer-Schwickerath next employed an improved carbon arc and finally the xenon arc lamp. In many of the first cases he treated, these light sources were used to produce chorioretinal adhesions surrounding retinal holes, particularly in the posterior pole.

Mention must also be made of Moran-Salas, who prior to Meyer-Schwickerath's investigations carried out a number of experiments with light photocoagulation in both rabbit and human eyes with limited success.[6]

DEVELOPMENT OF THE LASER

Theodore Maiman built the first laser, which employed a ruby crystal as medium, in July 1960.[7] In 1961, Zaret employed a ruby laser for iris and retinal photocoagulation in rabbits.[8] By 1963, Campbell and Koester as well as Zweng and his associates had each developed delivery systems for retinal photocoagulation employing the ruby laser.[9, 10] The ophthalmic ruby laser emitted pulses that lasted 600 microseconds and used a monocular direct ophthalmoscopic delivery system, as had the xenon arc photocoagulator. The ruby laser was used to treat retinal disorders, particularly retinal breaks. Beetham and Aiello used the ruby laser for peripheral fundus ablation in proliferative diabetic retinopathy—a precursor to argon laser panretinal photocoagulation.[11]

The ruby laser was a valuable tool, but it was quickly supplanted with the introduction of the argon laser photocoagulator. The earliest work in the development of an ophthalmic argon laser was done by L'Esperance and followed by the studies of Zweng, Little, Patz, and others.[12-14] The argon laser had several advantages over the ruby laser. Because the output was a steady continuous wave instead of a short pulse, it could be moved by existing fiberoptic technology into a slit lamp. This provided both a binocular microscopic delivery system, which made it possible to use a contact lens to visualize the peripheral fundus, and a more reliable means of controlling laser spot size. Moreover, because both melanin and hemoglobin have strong absorption coefficients for argon blue and green light, uniform and predictable treatment results were easier to obtain than with the ruby laser. Direct closure of vessels could be considered. Because the argon laser produced a continuous wave and not a pulsed output, long exposure times (typically 0.1 to 0.2 seconds) could be attained, compared with microsecond ruby pulses. As a result, peak power with the argon laser was much lower than with the ruby laser, another factor contributing to uniform and predictable photocoagulation.

The argon laser quickly became an integral part of modern ophthalmic therapy. National multicenter trials showed that argon panretinal photocoagulation was effective in decreasing the rate of visual loss in eyes of patients with proliferative diabetic retinopathy.[15] Other controlled trials showed that argon laser treatment was effective in decreasing visual loss in eyes of patients with choroidal neovascularization greater than 200 microns (μ) from the foveal center.[16]

A number of investigators studied the possibility of using argon or other lasers (in particular, short-pulsed ruby lasers) to create openings in the trabecular meshwork in eyes of patients with open angle glaucoma.[17, 18] Initial experiments in monkey eyes with the argon laser were generally unsuccessful and sometimes resulted in increases in intraocular pressure.[19] Despite these discouraging results, some ophthalmologists continued to consider other possibilities for laser therapy of open angle glaucoma. Wise and Witter devised a technique in which the argon laser was used to make nonpenetrating burns around the circumference of the trabecular meshwork.[20] This technique, which later was termed *laser trabeculoplasty,* has proved to be a major tool for the treatment of patients with open angle glaucoma.

THE DEVELOPMENT OF PHOTODISRUPTION

The development of ocular photodisruption is a remarkable chapter in the history of medicine and ophthalmology and illustrates the complex interaction of technologic innovation, clinical practice, and serendipity.

Photodisruption can be defined as the use of high peak power ionizing laser pulses to disrupt tissue. Light energy is concentrated in time and space to create optical breakdown—ionization of the target medium—with formation of a plasma, which is seen as a spark. The possibility of using optical radiation (as opposed to the discharge across two electrodes) to produce a plasma became a reality only after the development of lasers capable of emitting high power through very short light pulses. The first lasers built had output powers that were too low to produce optical breakdown. In 1962, Hellwarth developed the technique of Q-switching, which made it possible to create very brief "giant" ruby laser pulses delivered in 10 to 50 nanoseconds (nsec, billionths of a second) with maximum powers in the tens of megawatts.[21]

When a Q-switched ruby laser pulse is passed through a lens in air, a spark explodes at the focal point, exactly as in the electrical breakdown across a discharge gap. The first report of laser-induced spark formation was made in 1963 by Maker, Terhune, and Savage at the International Congress on Quantum

Electronics in Paris.[22] In the words of a contemporary observer, ". . .their report created a sensation. The laser spark phenomenon immediately, and for a long time, riveted the attention of physicists."[23] The discovery of the laser spark was the focus for the development of new experimental and theoretical studies in plasma physics for more than ten years.

Krasnov was the first to demonstrate that high peak power pulses could be used to produce clinically desirable disruption of ocular structures. In 1972, he reported use of a Q-switched ruby laser to treat the trabecular meshwork of eyes with open angle glaucoma.[24] He called the procedure *laser goniopuncture,* which produced a localized destruction of the trabecular meshwork and cyclodialysis. He described the procedure thus: "The effect of Q-switched laser goniopuncture is closely related to some phenomena observed in the angle as the procedure is being carried out. A very bright spark (plasma field formation) leaving a small gas bubble is seen at the target point. Sometimes, minute, crater-like defects with or without elevated margins are also visible."[25] To stress the relative importance of nonthermal acoustic mechanisms in producing these tissue effects, Krasnov coined the term *cold laser,* which is a misnomer, since plasma formation results in very localized temperature increases in excess of 10,000°C. Krasnov successfully ruptured the anterior lens capsule in rabbit eyes but was unable to do so in human eyes in which there was senile cataract. Subsequently, he reported a technique he called *phakopuncture* for the treatment of cataracts in young adults and children.[26] The anterior capsule was punctured at multiple pigmented sites to facilitate liquefaction and resorption of the lens material—a process that took up to one year. Because Krasnov's Q-switched ruby laser could not produce sufficient irradiance to disrupt the transparent anterior capsule, he treated the iris overlying the lens prior to the anterior capsule so as to produce pigment deposits in the anterior lens capsule. This procedure facilitated absorption of the ruby light energy and led to rupture of the capsule, presumably through a combination of thermal effects and optical breakdown.

Subsequent developments have shown that for a variety of technical reasons (such as the high order mode structure of the laser output, which increases the minimal spot size that can be achieved) the Q-switched ruby laser is not the optimal source for building a clinically practical ophthalmic photodisruptor. Nevertheless, Gaasterland did build a custom Q-switched ruby laser system that was successfully used for photodisruption. However, because the laser output could be brought only to a focal spot of 175 μ (as compared with 10 to 50 μ in current ophthalmic neodymium-yttrium-aluminum-garnet [Nd-YAG] photodisruptors), energies many times greater than necessary with current Nd-YAG photodisruptors were required for membranectomy. In addition, it was necessary to wait three minutes between laser shots, so the ruby rod could cool to allow subsequent shots to be reproducible in energy level. In November 1979, using this system, Gaasterland performed what was probably the first pulsed laser discission of a pupillary membrane done in the United States. Gaasterland described the treatment thus: "One application, at 65 millijoules, was delivered to the eye. This immediately created a linear rip of the membrane which slowly retracted into a round opening of approximately 2 mm. By the next day he had a pressure rise from the normal high teens to 46 mm Hg in this eye. Acetazolamide, pilocarpine, topical steroids and oral glycerine were all used during the next ten days to curb this response. By the end of that time, the pressure in the eye has returned to nearly normal."* The preoperative and postoperative appearance of this eye is depicted in Figure 1–2.

---

*Douglas E. Gaasterland: personal communication.

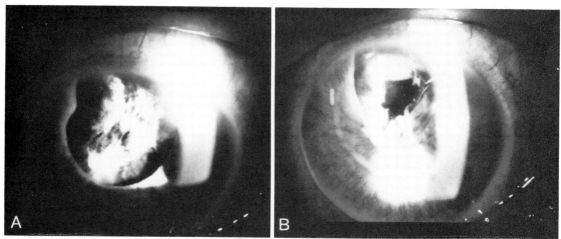

FIGURE 1–2   *(A)* Preoperative slit lamp photograph of the eye prior to photodisruption of the pupillary membrane. *(B)* Postoperative (30 minutes after treatment) appearance after membrane discission using a Q-switched ruby laser system. A single 65-mJ pulse application was used. (Courtesy of Douglas E. Gaasterland)

Several developments converged to make ophthalmic photodisruption a practical and highly desirable tool: the use of Q-switched and mode-locked neodymium lasers as laser sources, the pioneer clinical studies of Aron-Rosa and Fankhauser, and the growth of extracapsular cataract extraction and with it the need for later posterior capsulotomy. Fankhauser and his associates Van der Zypen, Bebie, and Loertscher worked first with Q-switched neodymium-glass and subsequently with Q-switched Nd-YAG lasers. They coupled a high-energy multimode industrial Nd-YAG laser to a slit lamp delivery system and performed experimental and clinical studies directed toward developing new techniques for glaucoma therapy. Although cyclodialysis clefts and trabeculo-puncture could be created in some eyes with a large reduction in intraocular pressure, the therapeutic effect was generally transient. Fankhauser performed clinical studies using his device for cutting a variety of intraocular mem-branes.[27–30] Aron-Rosa and her associate Griesemann worked with both Q-switched and mode-locked Nd-YAG lasers and chose the latter because the higher power densities possible with picosecond-long pulses permitted optical breakdown to be created more reliably than with the Q-switched laser that was available to them at that time.[31, 32] Aron-Rosa began her clinical trials in October 1978. She recognized the utility of Nd-YAG laser photodisruption for posterior capsulotomy following cataract extraction. In April 1981, at the annual meeting of the American Intraocular Implant Society she first reported her clinical results. This report marked the beginning of intense clinical and commercial interest in the development and utilization of Nd-YAG laser photodisruptors.

REFERENCES

1. Meyer-Schwickerath G. Light Coagulation. St Louis: C.V. Mosby, 1960, p 15.
2. Ibid., p 15.
3. Czerny. Ber. Wien. Acad. Wiss. 2:56, 1967. Cited by Meyer-Schwickerath, op. cit.
4. Deutschmann R. Ein experimenteller beitrag zur pathogense der sympathischen augen-entzundung. Albrecht Von Graefes Arch Klin Exp Ophthalmol 294–300, 1982.
5. Verhoeff EH, Bell L, Walker CB. The pathologic effects of radiant energy on the eye. Proc Am Acad Arts Sci 51:630–818, 1916.
6. Moran-Salas J. Arch Soc Oftal Hispano-Am 10:566, 1950.
7. Maiman TH. Stimulated optical radiation in ruby. Nature 187:493–7, 1960.

8. Zaret MM, Breinin GM, Schmidt H, Ripps H, Seigel IM, Solon LR. Ocular lesions produced an optical maser (laser). Science 134:1525–8, 1961.
9. Campbell CJ, Rittler MC, Koester CJ. The optical maser as retinal photocoagulator: An evaluation. Trans Am Acad Ophthalmol Otolaryngol 67:58–67, 1963.
10. Kapany NS, Peppers NA, Zweng HC, Flocks M. Retinal photocoagulation by lasers. Nature 199:146–9, 1963.
11. Beetham WP, Aiello LM, Balodimos M, Koncz L. Ruby laser photocoagulation of early diabetic neovascular retinopathy. Arch Ophthalmol 83:261–72, 1970.
12. L'Esperance FA Jr. An ophthalmic argon laser photocoagulation system: Design, construction, and laboratory investigations. Trans Am Ophthalmol Soc 66:827–904, 1968.
13. Little HL, Zweng HC, Peabody RR. Argon laser slit lamp retinal photocoagulation. Trans Am Acad Ophthalmol Otolaryngol 74:85–96, 1970.
14. Patz A, Maumenee AE, Ryan SJ. Argon laser photocoagulation. Trans Am Acad Ophthalmol Otolaryngol 75:569–79, 1971.
15. The Diabetic Retinopathy Study Research Group. Photocoagulation treatment of proliferative diabetic retinopathy: The second report of Diabetic Retinopathy Study findings. Ophthalmology 85:82–105, 1978.
16. Macular Photocoagulation Study Group. Argon laser photocoagulation for senile macular degeneration: Results of a randomized clinical trial. Arch Ophthalmol 100:912–8, 1982.
17. Krasnov M. Laseropuncture of anterior chamber angle in glaucoma. Am J Ophthalmol 75:674–8, 1973.
18. Wickham MG, Worthen DM. Argon laser trabeculotomy: Long-term follow-up. Trans Am Acad Ophthalmol Otolaryngol 86:495–503, 1979.
19. Gaasterland D, Kupfer C. Experimental glaucoma in the rhesus monkey. Invest Ophthalmol 13:455–7, 1974.
20. Wise JB, Witter SL. Argon laser therapy for open angle glaucoma. Arch Ophthalmol 97:319–22, 1979.
21. McClung FJ, Hellwarth RW. Giant optical pulsating from ruby. J Appl Phys 33:828–31, 1967.
22. Maker PD, Terhune RW, Savage CM. In Grivet, Bloembergen N (eds.). Quantum Electronics, Proceedings of the Third International Congress. New York: Columbia University Press, 1964, p 1559.
23. Raizer YP. Laser-Induced Discharge Phenomena. New York: Consultant Bureau, 1977, p 3.
24. Krasnov MM. Laser-puncture of the anterior chamber angle in glaucoma. Vestn Oftalmol 3:27–31, 1972.
25. Krasnov MM. Q-switched laser goniopuncture. Arch Ophthalmol 92:37–41, 1974.
26. Krasnov MM. Laser phakopuncture in the treatment of soft cataracts. Br J Ophthalmol 59:96–8, 1975.
27. Van der Zypen E, Bebie H, Fankhauser F. Morphologic studies about the efficiency of laser beams upon the structures of the angle of the anterior chamber. Int Ophthalmol 1,2:109–22, 1979.
28. Fankhauser F, Roussel P, Steffen J, Van der Zypen E, Chrenkova A. Clinical studies on the efficiency of a high power laser radiation upon some structures of the anterior segment of the eye. Int Ophthalmol 3:129–39, 1981.
29. Fankhauser F, Loertscher HP, Van der Zypen E. Clinical studies on high and lower power laser irradiation upon some structures of the anterior and posterior segments of the eye. Int Ophthalmol 5:15–32, 1982.
30. Fankhauser F, Van der Zypen E. Future of the laser in ophthalmology. Trans Ophthal Soc UK 102:159–63, 1982.
31. Aron-Rosa D, Aron J, Greisemann J, Thyzel R. Use of the neodymium YAG laser to open the posterior capsule after lens implant surgery: A preliminary report. J Am Intraocul Implant Soc 6:352–4, 1980.
32. Aron-Rosa D. Use of a pulsed neodymium-YAG laser for anterior capsulotomy before extracapsular extraction. J Am Intraocul Implant Soc 7:332–3, 1981.

2
LASER FUNDAMENTALS

PROPERTIES OF LASER LIGHT

Lasers are only one of many sources of light energy. The unique properties of laser light, however, make laser-emitted light particularly suitable for many medical applications. These properties are monochromaticity, directionality, coherence, polarization, and intensity.

Lasers emit light at only one wavelength or sometimes at a combination of several wavelengths that can be separated easily. Thus a "pure" or *monochromatic* beam is obtained. Although the wavelength spread is not infinitely small, a gas laser emission line can be as narrow as 0.01 nanometers (nanometer [nm] = 10^{-9} meter), compared with the wavelengths over a 300 nm span that occur in white light. At best, a filter might reduce the transmission of white light to a color range (band width) of 5 nm. From a medical viewpoint, coloration of light can be used to enhance absorption or transmission by a target tissue with a certain absorption spectrum. The wavelength specificity of a laser greatly exceeds the absorption specificity of pigments in tissues. Another useful property of monochromaticity is that chromatic aberration in lens systems cannot occur. Thus monochromatic light can be focused to a smaller spot than can white light.

The second property of laser-emitted light is *directionality*. Lasers emit a narrow beam that spreads very slowly. As is explained later in this chapter, lasers amplify only those photons that travel along a very narrow path between two mirrors. This process serves as a very efficient mechanism for collimating light. Beam divergence is the physical measurement of the directionality of the light beam leaving the laser. Divergence is usually expressed in milliradians (mrad). It should be recalled that 2π radians is 360 degrees. A typical laser has a beam divergence of 1 mrad, which indicates that the beam increases by about 1 mm in diameter for every meter traveled. Directionality makes it easy to collect all of the light energy in a simple lens system and to focus this light to a small spot.

Coherence is the term most often associated with lasers. The degree of coherence is the extent to which the electromagnetic field of the light wave varies regularly and predictably in time and space. Laser light projected onto a rough surface has a characteristic sparkling quality known as *laser speckle*. This phenomenon occurs because the irregular reflection of highly coherent light creates irregular interference patterns, or speckle. Coherence of laser light is utilized to create the interference fringes of the ophthalmic diagnostic laser

11

interferometer. In therapeutic ophthalmic lasers coherency, like directionality, is important because of the improved focusing characteristics.

Many lasers emit linearly polarized light. *Polarization* is another aspect of coherency. Polarization is incorporated in the laser system to allow maximum transmission through the laser medium without loss caused by reflection. The specific polarization of the light beam is not currently utilized in medical applications. However, the most commonly employed electro-optical Q-switches work by manipulation of polarized windows in the beam path.

In most medical applications, the most important property of lasers is brightness or *intensity*. Radiometry is the measurement of electromagnetic radiation. Radiant energy is measured in joules (J), and radiant power (or "flux") is measured in watts (W). The reader should recall that energy is work and power is the rate at which work is done. One joule = 1 watt × 1 second or 1 W = 1 J/sec. *Intensity* is the power in a beam of a given angular size, and *brightness* is the intensity per unit area. In medical laser applications, the four important radiometric terms are *energy* (J), *power* (W), *radiant energy density* (J/cm^2), and *irradiance* (W/cm^2) (Table 2–1). The laser output is quantitated in either joules or watts. The tissue effect is then determined by the focal point spot size, which determines energy density and irradiance (or, less properly stated, "power density"). In ophthalmic lasers, spot size is conventionally given as the diameter. Thus a 50-micron (μ) spot size has an area of π $(25 \times 10^{-4})^2$ cm^2, or about 2×10^{-5} cm^2.

In an ophthalmic laser with a continuous beam of light, such as a laser using argon and krypton, the control panel meter gives the power in watts, whereas in a pulsed laser, such as the Nd-YAG laser, the meter reading gives the energy per pulse in joules. This specification is convenient because the continuous laser beam has a constant power, but the energy varies according to the shutter setting (for example, 100 mW for 0.2 seconds delivers 20 mJ). In the case of pulsed lasers, the beam is intermittent, and thus there is both average and peak power. In a single discrete pulse, however, there is a determinate amount of energy that can be readily measured. Knowledge of two of the variables of energy, power, and time allows ready calculation of the third variable.

In sum, directionality, polarization, coherence, and to some degree monochromaticity enhance the most important characteristic of lasers, which is brightness. The sun has a power of 10^{26} watts but emits energy in all directions at a great distance from the earth. Thus, a simple 1 mW helium neon laser is 100 times brighter than the sun. Combined with the ability of monochromaticity to target selected tissues and to avoid others on the basis of spectral absorption, lasers are a unique tool in medicine. This is particularly true in ophthalmology, since the eye is designed to allow light transmission to most of its structures. Figure 2–1 summarizes the major properties of laser light in comparison with a conventional light source.

TABLE 2–1. RADIOMETRIC TERMINOLOGY FOR MEDICAL LASERS

Term	Unit
Radiant energy	joule*
Radiant power	watt
Radiant energy density	joules/cm^2
Irradiance	watts/cm^2
Radiant intensity	watts/sterad†
Radiance (brightness)	watts/sterad cm^2

*1 joule = 1 watt × 1 sec.
†Steradian is the unit of solid angle. There are 4 π steradians in a sphere.

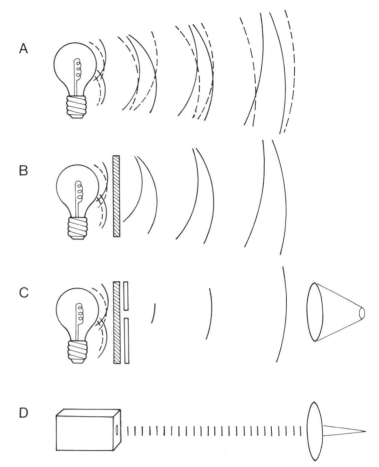

FIGURE 2–1

Comparison of properties of incandescent and laser light sources. *(A)* The incandescent bulb emits incoherent rapidly divergent light with a broad mixture of wavelengths (solid and broken waves). *(B)* A narrow band pass filter absorbs all but a narrow portion of the spectrum (solid waves) but consequently absorbs much of the light energy. *(C)* Directionality and coherency are improved with the addition of a pinhole aperture, but further energy is lost; a lens system collects some of the light and brings it to a focus. *(D)* A laser emits monochromatic, directional, coherent light that is readily collected by a lens system and brought to a much smaller focal area. Compared with the incandescent source, the power and irradiance of the laser system are many orders of magnitude greater.

ELEMENTS OF A LASER

All ophthalmic lasers currently in use require three basic elements: (1) an *active medium* that emits coherent radiation, (2) a means of energy input known as *pumping,* and (3) the opportunity for oscillation and amplification through optical *feedback. LASER* is an acronym for Light Amplification by Stimulated Emission of Radiation—a term that highlights the key event that creates laser light, which is *stimulated emission.*

In 1917 Albert Einstein explained the mathematical relationships of three atomic transition processes: *stimulated absorption, spontaneous emission,* and *stimulated emission.* According to the fundamental principles of quantum physics, certain atomic energy transitions are highly probable or "allowed." Light energy can readily induce such an allowed transition, causing the energy of the atom to move from its ground state (E_0) to an excited state (E_1). The atom absorbs a quantum of energy at a predictable frequency appropriate to cause the specific transition.* If the source of illumination were white light, a discrete frequency would be subtracted (line spectra) from the illuminating beam. Each atomic element has a characteristic line spectrum. This process is known as stimulated absorption (Fig. 2–2*A*).

---

*Recall that $E = h\nu = hc/\lambda$, where energy *(E)* and frequency *(ν)* are related by Planck's constant *(h),* and frequency and wavelength *(λ)* are inversely related by the relationship $\nu = c/\lambda$. *c* is the speed of light, 3×10^8m/sec.

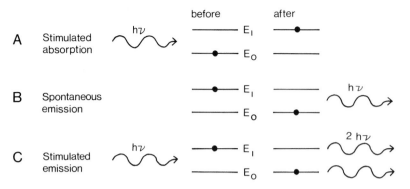

FIGURE 2–2

Schematic representation of an electron moving between the lowest energy (ground) state (E_0) and an allowed excited state (E_1) in conjunction with absorption of a quantum of light energy $(\Delta E = E_1 - E_0 = h\nu)$. *(A)* Stimulated absorption, *(B)* spontaneous emission, and *(C)* stimulated emission are demonstrated.

Because the lowest energy state is the most stable, the excited atom soon emits a quantum of energy at the same frequency in order to return to the ground state. This process can occur without external stimulation (*spontaneous emission,* Fig. 2–2*B*) or in conjunction with further stimulation by another quantum of light at the same transition frequency (*stimulated emission,* Fig. 2–2*C*). Radiation emitted by spontaneous emission occurs randomly in time, whereas radiation emitted by stimulated emission is in phase with the stimulating wave. Therefore, stimulated emission is coherent. After stimulated absorption the majority of energy release is through spontaneous emission occurring incoherently in all directions, and only a small fraction of the energy is normally released as coherent stimulated emission. The laser environment, however, amplifies only the stimulated emission.

The *active medium* is an atomic environment that supports stimulated emission. The active medium allows a large number of atoms to be energized above the ground state, so that stimulated emission may occur. The particular atomic energy transition determines the wavelength of the emission ($E = h\nu = hc/\lambda$). Lasers are usually named for the active medium. The medium can be a gas (argon, krypton, carbon dioxide, or helium with neon), a liquid (dye), a solid (an active element supported by a crystal, such as neodymium supported by yttrium-aluminum-garnet [Nd-YAG] and erbium supported by yttrium-lan-thanum-fluoride [Er-YLF]), or a semiconductor.

The second requirement for a laser is the provision of a means of energy input to the active medium such that a majority of the atoms are in an energy state higher than the ground state. This condition is known as a *population inversion,* because it is the inverse of the usual condition in which the majority of atoms are in the lowest or ground energy state. The energy input that creates the population inversion is known as *pumping.* Gas lasers are usually pumped by electrical discharge between electrodes in the gas; dye lasers are often pumped by other lasers; and solid crystals are usually pumped by incoherent light such as the xenon arc flash lamp.

The final requirement, once population inversion in an active medium has been achieved, is for a means of *optical feedback* to promote stimulated emission and suppress spontaneous emission. The laser cavity is an optical resonator providing an environment that creates this optical feedback. Mirrors are placed at each end of a beam path to cause reflected light to pass back and forth through the active medium, in which the pump maintains a population inversion (Fig. 2–3). Thus a light wave resonates through the active medium and each time increases the total coherent light energy through stimulated emission. Spontaneous emission, which occurs randomly in all directions, rarely strikes a mirror and therefore is not amplified.

The last element in this elementary laser design is a mechanism for releasing

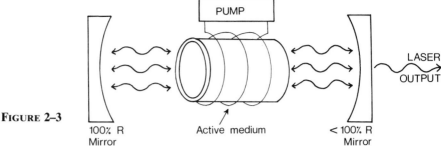

FIGURE 2–3

100% R
Mirror

Active medium

< 100% R
Mirror

Elementary laser schematic illustrating the active medium within the optical resonant cavity formed by the mirrors, and the pump, which creates a population inversion in the active medium. One mirror is fully reflective (100 per cent R), while the other mirror is partially transparent (< 100 per cent R). As schematically drawn, the mirror is 66 per cent reflective, and the average light wave makes three round trips through the active medium before being emitted.

some of the oscillating laser light from the cavity. This is achieved by making one of the mirrors fully reflective and the other mirror only partially reflective. A portion of the light waves striking this second mirror leaves the cavity as the emitted laser beam. The reflectivity of the mirror is selected to satisfy the requirements for efficient amplification in a particular system. For example, if a laser has a 98 per cent reflective mirror, the light waves are coherently amplified by stimulated emission during an average of 50 round trips through the active medium before they are emitted as the laser beam.

LASER SOURCES

Solid-state laser sources commonly used in medical applications are ruby and neodymium-YAG. Argon, krypton, and carbon dioxide are the most important gas laser sources used in medicine. A variety of new laser sources has been developed in the past decade, some of which hold promise for medical application. In 1975, it was shown that rare gas atoms in metastable excited states could react with halogens to form diatomic rare gas halides in a bound excited (excimer) state. Decay of these excimer molecules to a weakly bound or unbound ground state is accompanied by emission of a photon with ultraviolet frequency. Excimer lasers efficiently produce high-power ultraviolet irradiation. A number of different excimer molecules can be created, and each is associated with a specific transition and emission wavelength: ArF (193 nm), KrF (249 nm), and XeF (351 nm). As is discussed in Chapter 4, these lasers hold particular promise as tools for tissue ablation. Alexandrite is another new laser source—the most highly developed member of a new class of tunable solid-state laser sources. Alexandrite is pumped by flash lamp and is continuously tunable over the range 700 to 820 nm, with average output powers in excess of 100 W. With the use of doubling crystals and other nonlinear wavelength shifting techniques, an alexandrite laser could generate wavelengths from the ultraviolet to the midinfrared ranges.

THE LASER OUTPUT

Laser Modes. In a real laser cavity, the resonating waves consist of a large number of waves, with each traveling in slightly different directions between

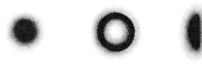

TEM$_{00}$ MODE   TEM$_{01}$* MODE   TEM$_{01}$ MODE

FIGURE 2–4

Three examples of transverse electromagnetic modes, designated TEM$_{mn}$, as photographed in an expanding beam. The fundamental mode is designated TEM$_{00}$. (Courtesy of Spectra-Physics Inc.)

the two end mirrors. The result is a three-dimensional electromagnetic field pattern of resonant modes that can be mathematically described. The different modes are designated by the notation TEM$_{mnq}$. TEM stands for Transverse Electro-Magnetic, meaning that the electrical and magnetic fields are each perpendicular, or transverse, to the direction of propagation of the light beam. The subscript q designates the *axial mode* of the laser. Axial modes are discussed later with regard to mode-locking. The number q is of little interest and is usually omitted. The subscripts m and n designate the *transverse mode* of the laser beam. Thus a given transverse mode is designated TEM$_{mn}$. Figure 2–4 illustrates several different transverse modes, which can be recorded on light-sensitive paper exposed to the expanding beam. The transverse modes are "hot spots" of light of higher intensity. The number of transverse modes depends on many variables in laser design, particularly mirror size and shape.

The higher-order transverse modes have larger beam divergence than the fundamental mode, TEM$_{00}$ (often referred to as *mono-mode* in the European literature). Thus TEM$_{00}$ has the lowest beam divergence and allows the laser beam to be focused to the smallest possible spot, which is particularly important for ophthalmic short-pulsed Nd-YAG lasers. Generally, nonfundamental modes are suppressed by the placement of an aperture within the laser cavity, as illustrated in Figure 2–5. Of course, the energy that is contained in the nonfundamental transverse modes is lost. If an adjustable iris diaphragm aperture is employed, then the fundamental mode may be selected when the smallest focal spot is required, and the aperture can be opened and higher-order modes allowed for applications in which higher total power is more important than higher power density (irradiance).

The border of any light beam, even in the fundamental mode, is not sharp and discrete. Rather, the power distribution in the fundamental mode has a bell-shaped distribution. The mathematical equation for TEM$_{mn}$ reduces, for TEM$_{00}$, to what is known as a *Gaussian*. A Gaussian spatial distribution is diagramed in Figure 2–6 along with the defining equation.* The $1/e$ points include 63 per cent of the total power, while the $1/e^2$ points include 86.5 per cent of the total power.

---

*I_{00} *(r)* $= e^{-2r^2/w^2}$ where I = irradiance at a given radius *(r)* from the optical axis, and w is the unfocused spot size of the beam as it leaves the laser. The *beam spot size* is defined as the point at which the beam intensity is $1/e^2$ of its peak value on the optical axis ($w = r$, and thus $I_{00} = e^{-2} = 1/e^2$).

FIGURE 2–5

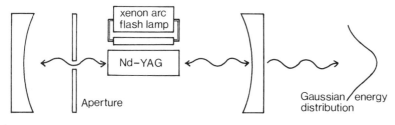

xenon arc flash lamp

Nd–YAG

Aperture

Gaussian energy distribution

Schematic representation of an Nd-YAG laser cavity containing an aperture designed to suppress all transverse modes except the fundamental mode, TEM$_{00}$, which has a Gaussian spatial distribution.

FIGURE 2–6

A fundamental mode laser beam does not have a sharp border, but rather a smooth exponential decline in spatial intensity from a maximum at the center. The mathematical expression of this Gaussian distribution is $I = e^{-2r^2/w^2}$. The relative intensity at the center ($r = 0$) is 1.

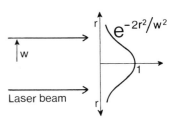

Gaussian beams can be focused to the minimal spot size because they progagate uniformly (that is, they maintain the Gaussian distribution as the beam travels through space) and because the same phase is present across the wave front (the beam is "uniphase"). An ideal beam can achieve a minimal focal spot radius r predicted by the equation $r = \lambda L/2\pi a$, where λ is the wavelength of light, L is the focal length of the lens, and a is the radius of the lens transmitting the beam. An alternative expression is $r = \lambda f/\pi$, where $f = L/2a$, the f-number of the lens system, as used in cameras. For example, a commercial ophthalmic Nd-YAG laser delivered through a slit lamp typically may have a solid cone angle of 16 degrees, which calculates to an f-number of about 3.6. With a wavelength of 1064 (1064×10^{-9} m) the minimum spot radius is therefore 1.2 μ, giving a minimum diameter of 2.4 μ under ideal conditions. The importance of minimizing focal spot size to maximize irradiance is made evident in the discussion of optical breakdown in Chapter 3.

Axial modes or *longitudinal modes* are the frequencies at which the laser cavity is resonant. It should be recalled that in the laser cavity light waves are amplified as they pass back and forth between the two mirrors. The wave and its reflections must be in phase in order that the electric fields summate rather than cancel each other. The length of the cavity therefore must be equal to an integral number of half-wavelengths.* The two nearest resonant axial mode frequencies can also be determined. For a typical laser with a cavity 25 cm long, the separation of resonant frequencies is 600 megahertz.† Because laser transitions are much broader than this, there can be many axial modes in a laser line width.

Mode-Locking. The reader should recall that power is energy divided by time. To obtain high power, energy can be increased to its maximum. Practical design considerations limit the total energy output. The alternative method of obtaining high power, which achieves much higher peak power than can be obtained purely through increased energy, is by reduction of the time over which the energy is delivered. The two principal means of compressing the laser output in time to achieve high peak power are known as *Q-switching* and *mode-locking*.

Mode-locking takes advantage of the axial modes discussed previously. Three conditions are necessary. First, the laser medium must have a sufficiently broad transition to create a large number of oscillating axial modes. Second, the cavity should be relatively long so that the separation between modes is small. Third, there must be a mechanism for synchronizing phase relationships.

The process of mode-locking is similar to the audible summation of musical tones with nearby frequencies, called "beating," which is heard as a periodic

---

*$L = q(\lambda/2)$, where L is the length of the cavity and q is an integer (the same q as in TEM_{mnq}). q represents the number of wavelengths in the cavity that are resonant. For example, if the wavelength is 1000 nm (1000×10^{-9}m) and the cavity is 25 cm long, $q = 5 \times 10^5$.

†Frequency $\nu = c/\lambda$. By substitution in $L = q(\lambda/2)$, it is found that the frequency difference $\Delta\nu$ between q and $q+1$ is $\Delta\nu = c/2L$, where c is the speed of light, 3×10^{10} cm/sec. Thus for a 25-cm cavity $\Delta\nu = 6 \times 10^8$ sec^{-1} = 600 MHz, so there is a separation between two resonant wavelengths of approximately 0.0002 nm.

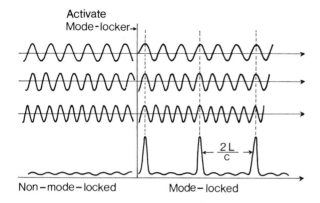

FIGURE 2–7

Three axial modes with random phase *(left)* are brought into phase with use of a mode-locker *(right)*. The result is an output beam with periodic high peak power pulses, spaced $2L/c$ apart. (After O'Shea, Callen, and Rhodes)

surge in intensity. In the case of a musical instrument, the phase relationships are synchronized by the musical instrument. In lasers, the phase relationships are synchronized by a shutter. The shutter is placed close to one of the cavity mirrors. The shutter may be electro-optic or acousto-optic (as discussed further under Q-switching), in which case the shutter mechanism is called *active mode-locking.* In ophthalmic applications the most common shutter is a saturable dye, called *passive mode-locking* (more accurately, Q-switched mode-locking, but the term Q-switch is usually omitted). The dye has the property of absorbing low-power light pulses, but the dye bleaches and becomes transparent on exposure to high-power light pulses. When the dye bleaches, the high-power pulses are reflected and amplified. In this manner, the axial modes become synchronized or mode-locked. The dye must be able to alternately bleach and recover opacity within picoseseconds (psec, 10^{-12} seconds).

In Figure 2–7 the summations of non-mode-locked and mode-locked axial modes are compared. The mode-locked phases periodically summate at a time interval equal to the time for a round trip of light in the cavity.*

Q-Switching. The other principal mechanism for attaining high peak power also occurs through an intracavity shutter called a Q-switch. In addition to the Q-switch itself, the other necessary condition for high peak power is an active medium that allows atoms to remain in the high-energy state for a relatively long time. Solid-state media (such as Nd-YAG and ruby) are particularly suitable in this regard.

Figure 2–8 illustrates the generation of Q-switched pulse. The Q-switch shutter is initially closed, or opaque, so that one of the mirrors is optically "removed" from the cavity, and oscillation cannot occur. The flash lamp fires, and a large population inversion occurs. Because oscillation cannot occur, losses are limited to spontaneous emission; stimulated emission and amplification are prevented. Maximum energy or "gain" is thus placed in the laser medium.

At the appropriate moment the Q-switch shutter is opened, and the mirror is exposed. Oscillation and stimulated emission then rapidly occur, with emission of a single short high-power pulse.

There are a number of methods of Q-switching, including the use of rotating mirrors, saturable dyes, and acousto-optic modulators. The latter mechanism uses sound waves to cause diffraction of light. The most common Q-switch, however, is an electro-optic modulator known as a Pockel's cell that applies voltage across a crystal to vary polarization. Polarity can be changed

---

*This interval is $2L/c$. Ophthalmic mode-locked lasers often have pulse spacing of 5 nsec. Cavity length L is thus $(5 \times 10^{-9}$ sec) $(3 \times 10^{10}$ cm/sec$)/2 = 75$ cm.

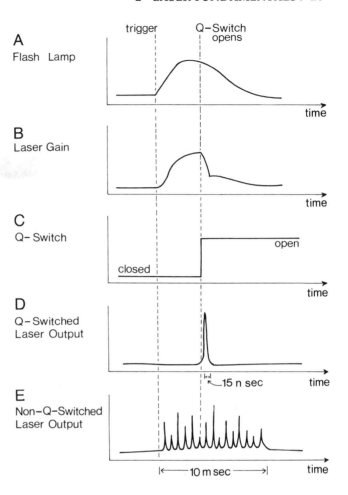

A
Flash Lamp

B
Laser Gain

C
Q-Switch

D
Q-Switched
Laser Output

E
Non-Q-Switched
Laser Output

FIGURE 2–8

Generation of a Q-switched pulse. The horizontal axis represents time. *(A)* The flash lamp fires typically over an interval of 10 to 20 msec. When laser gain is maximal *(B)* the Q-switch opens *(C)*, and a pulse of high peak power is emitted with a typical duration between 2 and 30 nsec *(D)*. If the Q-switch had been open throughout the flash lamp pulse, an irregular low-power laser emission would occur over the duration of adequate energy input from the flash lamp *(E)*. The vertical scales in *(D)* and *(E)*, representing power, are different by many orders of magnitude, with a Q-switched power of 100,000 W and a non-Q-switched power of 100 W.

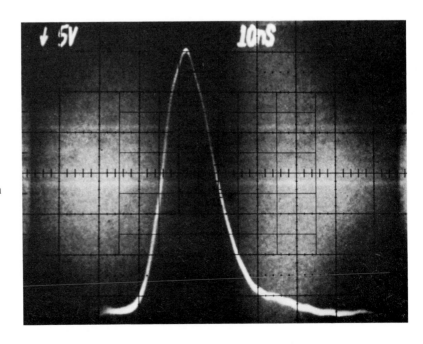

FIGURE 2–9

Oscilloscopic tracing of a single Q-switched Nd-YAG laser pulse with a pulse width of 15 nsec.

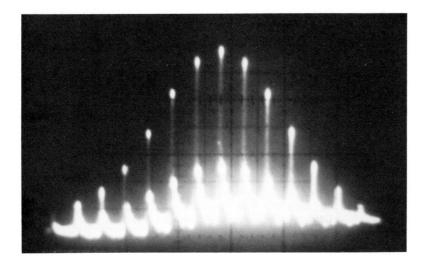

FIGURE 2–10

Oscilloscopic tracing of a train of mode-locked Nd-YAG laser pulses with 5 nsec interpulse spacing. Each pulse has a width of 30 psec, which cannot be resolved by the oscilloscope.

rapidly by 90 degrees, which makes the cell either transparent or opaque to the polarized laser beam.

The *Q* in the term Q-switch stands for the *quality factor** of the laser cavity, which is defined as the energy stored in the cavity divided by the energy lost per cycle. Thus the Q-switch changes the quality factor of the cavity from a high Q to a low Q with rapid extraction of high power.

Figure 2–9 is a photograph of an oscilloscope tracing of a single Q-switched pulse, and Figure 2–10 is a photograph of a train of mode-locked pulses, both from a Nd-YAG laser. A typical single Q-switched pulse has a duration between 2 and 30 nsec. A typical mode-locked pulse train consists of seven to 10 pulses spaced over a total of 35 to 50 nsec. The oscilloscope is too slow to resolve each picosecond-long pulse, but indirect measurement techniques reveal a typical pulse width of 30 psec. Thus the average individual mode-locked pulse is 500 times shorter than a 15 nsec Q-switched pulse and for the same total

---

*$Q = 2 \times$ energy stored ÷ energy dissipated per cycle.

TABLE 2–2. COMPARISON OF FOUR TYPICAL LASER TIME REGIMES AND ENERGY AND POWER RELATIONSHIPS EMPLOYED IN CLINICAL OPHTHALMOLOGY

	Continuous-Wave (CW) Argon	Long-Pulsed Nd-YAG	Q-Switched Nd-YAG	Mode-Locked Nd-YAG
Individual pulse duration	select 0.1 sec	10 msec	15 nsec	30 psec
Wavelength (nm)	488 514	1064	1064	1064
Energy (mJ)	100	1000	2	2
Power (W)	1	100	1.3×10^5	6.7×10^6 (per pulse)
Assigned spot diameter (μ)	50	50	50	50
Irradiance (W/cm²)	5.1×10^4	5.0×10^6	6.6×10^9	3.4×10^{11} (per pulse)

energy has 50 to 100 times the peak power. Current ophthalmic Q-switched Nd-YAG lasers have a maximum output of 10 to 20 mJ, while mode-locked units have a maximum output of approximately 4.5 mJ. Table 2–2 compares the energy and power relationships at clinical levels between four ophthalmic lasers illustrating the four major classes of laser temporal output: continuous-wave (*cw*), long-pulsed (milli- to microsecond), short-pulsed Q-switched, and mode-locked lasers. Because of the extremely short pulse length, the short-pulsed YAG laser, with 50 times less energy than an argon laser pulse, can produce power densities greater than a billion watts per sq cm compared with 50 thousand watts per sq cm for the argon laser. The picosecond-long pulse is roughly 10 billion times shorter than a typical argon application. This is comparable with the difference between the thickness of ten pages of this book and the width of the United States of America. During the duration of a 30-psec pulse, light travels 9 mm in space; during a 0.1-second argon pulse, light travels three quarters of the distance around the Earth.

REFERENCES

1. O'Shea DC, Callen WR, Rhodes WT. Introduction to Lasers and Their Applications. Reading, MA: Addison-Wesley, 1977.
2. Ready JF. Effects of High-Power Laser Radiation. New York: Academic Press, 1971.

3

OPTICAL BREAKDOWN, PLASMA FORMATION, AND PHOTODISRUPTION

When a target is heated by absorbing light energy, the effect is proportionate to the cause. It is *linear*: more light produces more heat. *Nonlinear* effects are sudden all-or-nothing phenomena. While the linear effect of heating by light energy is familiar as it occurs in sunlight, nonlinear light phenomena are less common. Optical breakdown is a nonlinear effect achieved when laser light is sufficiently condensed in time and space to achieve high irradiance or density of power. Optical breakdown is a sudden event that is visibly manifested by a spark and accompanied by an audible snap, with dramatic damage to a target. When focused to a small spot, usually less than 50 microns (μ) in diameter, Q-switched and mode-locked Nd-YAG lasers can produce adequate irradiance to induce optical breakdown.

The most common everyday examples of this nonlinear process are lightning and, on a smaller scale, electrical sparks. In these instances, electrical charges build, which is to say that an electromagnetic field grows in strength, until enough power is present to accelerate electrons into complete dissociation from their atoms. The atmosphere becomes ionized and can conduct electrons to ground. This process lowers the electromagnetic field strength; the electrons rejoin with the positively charged atoms; and the event is complete. The visible bluish white lightning or spark is the energy released as light energy or photons when the electrons rejoin their atoms. The audible thunder or snap is our perception of the pressure wave created by this sudden ionization process.

Physicists call this ionized state a *plasma*. In a plasma, electrons have freely dissociated from their atoms, which then become positive ions in a process that occurs in the presence of photons. Thus a plasma can conduct electricity, like a metal, but in most other properties plasma behaves like a gas. Plasma is properly considered a fourth state of matter, along with solids, liquids, and gas, in a manner analogous with the ancient belief in four fundamental elements of earth, water, air, and fire.[1]

Plasma can be created by heat, electricity, or radiant energy, such as laser light. While plasmas seem uncommon on the relatively cool planet Earth, two common examples have already been mentioned, those of lightning and electrical sparks. Additional examples are neon signs, the ionosphere in the outer Earth atmosphere, which reflects radio waves, and the aurora bourealis or northern lights. The sun, and in fact all stars, is made completely of plasma, and thus 90 per cent of the universe is plasma.[1] Plasma is thus the most common state of matter!

OPTICAL BREAKDOWN AND PLASMA FORMATION

Light energy can create plasma when high irradiance is achieved, commonly between 10^{10} and 10^{12} watts per sq cm (W/cm^2). This process of optical breakdown was demonstrated in gas when Q-switched lasers capable of reaching levels of high irradiance became available.[2] The level of Q-switched laser irradiance necessary for initiating optical breakdown has an electrical field strength in excess of 10^7 volts per cm (V/cm). Figure 3–1 summarizes the processes by which Q-switched and mode-locked lasers lead to photodisruption.

Initiation. Two different mechanisms are responsible for optical breakdown by Q-switched and mode-locked Nd-YAG lasers, because of the effect of pulse duration.[3, 4] Q-switched pulses of several nanoseconds' duration cause ionization, mainly by focal heating of the target. This is termed *thermionic emission.*[5] At the focal spot, temperatures in excess of several thousand degrees Celsius are achieved. Impurities in the target enhance this process.

Mode-locked pulses typically lasting 20 to 30 psec have a different dominant mechanism to initiate ionization, *multiphoton absorption.* Each photon at 1064 nm from a Nd-YAG laser has an energy quantum of 1.17 electron volts (eV), but many atoms require 10 eV or more to be ionized. Thus multiple photons must be absorbed to adequately accelerate the electron to achieve ionization.[6]

These two initiation mechanisms are shown in Figure 3–1*B.* The longer Q-switched pulse does not have adequate electrical field strength to initiate ionization by multiphoton absorption and depends on heating enhanced by focal impurity for the initiation ionization.[7, 8]

Growth. Whether initiation is by thermionic emission or multiphoton absorption, once the starting free electrons (the so-called "lucky electrons") have been generated, plasma grows through the mechanism of *electron avalanche* or *cascade.* A free electron absorbs a photon and accelerates.* The accelerated electron strikes another atom and ionizes it, resulting in two free electrons each with less individual energy. These two free electrons, in turn, absorb more photons, accelerate, strike other atoms, and release two more electrons, and so forth, as shown in Figure 3–1*C.*[7-9] The process of photon absorption and electron acceleration in the presence of an atom or ion is technically known as *inverse bremsstrahlung.*†[10]

For plasma to grow, the irradiance must be intense enough to cause rapid ionization, such that losses do not quench the electron avalanche. Inelastic collisions and free-electron diffusion from the focal volume are the main mechanisms of loss during avalanche ionization.[11, 12]

The threshold for optical breakdown is higher for mode-locked picosecond-long pulses than for Q-switched nanosecond-long pulses.[3, 4] In air, the threshold for a single 25-psec pulse is 10^{14} W/cm^2 compared with a threshold for a 10-nsec pulse of 10^{11} W/cm^2. In ophthalmic Nd-YAG mode-locked lasers, the laser delivers a train of seven to ten 25-psec pulses each spaced 5 nsec apart. The

---

Photon absorption technically is energy transfer to the free electron when the electric field of the laser light accelerates the electron.

†The term *inverse bremsstrahlung* refers to the physical principle that in order to conserve momentum the acceleration of the electron must take place in the field of a heavy particle (atom, molecule, or ion) that recoils.

FIGURE 3–1

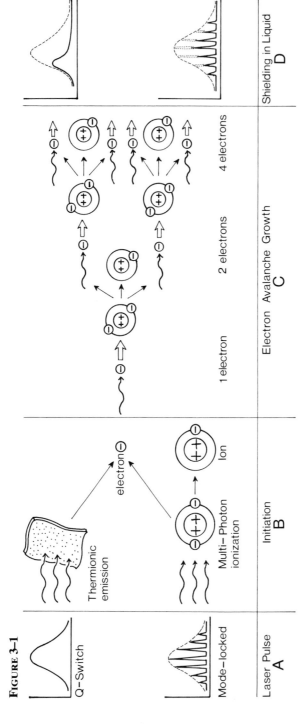

Initiation, growth, and shielding effect of plasma formation by optical breakdown. The dominant mechanism of initiation of ionization by a Q-switched pulse is thermionic emission and by a mode-locked pulse is multiphoton absorption (*B*). After a free electron has been produced, the plasma grows as a cascade or avalanche when photons (⌇) cause free electrons (⊝) to accelerate (⇒) and collide with atoms. This collision results in more free electrons and ions (*C*). The photon absorption reduces light transmission along the beam path, compared with the original pulse shape (*A*), in a process known as shielding (*D*).

total energy delivered in achieving optical breakdown is ultimately the same for a single Q-switched pulse and a train of mode-locked pulses,[13, 14] although the peak power of the picosecond-long pulse must be, on the average, about 100 to 1000 times higher than the Q-switched pulse to cause avalanche ionization.

These time-dependent differences in initiation mechanisms explain some observations of differences between the clinical Q-switched and mode-locked lasers. The presence of impurities in the target greatly enhances thermionic ionization but has little effect on multiphoton ionization. Thus there is greater variability in achieving optical breakdown with a Q-switched laser when it is working near threshold.[7, 8] At near-threshold levels, Q-switched breakdown is perceived as being more explosive, because for nanosecond-long pulses the irradiance necessary for thermionic initiation is greater than the irradiance necessary for plasma growth. Q-switched avalanche ionization is therefore precipitous once initiation occurs.[15] The closer match of the irradiance requirement for picosecond-long pulse initiation and growth makes the threshold effect smaller and less explosive for the mode-locked laser.

Plasma Shielding. Once formed, plasma absorbs and scatters incident light. This property "shields" underlying structures that are in the beam path. Light absorption by the plasma occurs through the same mechanism as does plasma growth, namely by inverse bremsstrahlung. Incident light energy is absorbed by further electron acceleration. Figure 3–1 *A* and *D* illustrate the alteration in the transmitted Q-switched and mode-locked pulse profiles.

Considerable confusion has been engendered by claims regarding the importance of plasma shielding in retinal protection during anterior segment use of the ophthalmic Nd-YAG laser and by purported differences in shielding

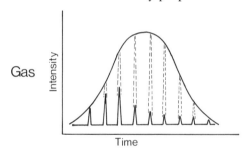
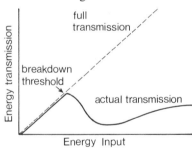

Gas

FIGURE 3–2

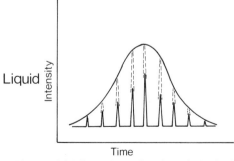
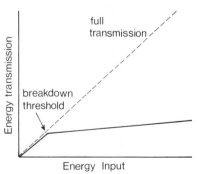

Liquid

Plasma shielding of a train of mode-locked pulses by breakdown in a gas *(top)* and liquid *(bottom)*. The plasma persists between pulses in the gas, but not in the liquid. The result is enhanced shielding and a protective decrease in energy transmission for suprathreshold pulses in the gas. Because liquid is very dense compared with gas, the breakdown threshold is lower, but the plasma lifetime is shorter than the interpulse spacing, and the transmission curve does not drop in liquid as it does in gas.

between Q-switched and mode-locked lasers. Retinal protection is discussed in detail in Chapter 4; suffice it to say that the beam divergence after the focal point, determined by the optics of the delivery system, can be made adequate to protect the retina in the absence of any plasma shielding.[16]

No significant difference has been demonstrated between plasma shielding by mode-locked and by Q-switched scientific and ophthalmic Nd-YAG lasers when targets of physiologic saline solution, hyaluronic acid, and a membrane in physiologic saline solution have been tested.[14, 17] When the target is a gas, a train of mode-locked pulses shows enhanced shielding compared with a single Q-switched pulse, because in a gas the plasma persists longer than the pulse spacing in a typical mode-locked train with 5-nsec interpulse spacing. The initial pulses create the plasma, which then persists and heavily shields subsequent pulses in the train.[13, 18] Thus absolute light transmission drops after the threshold for optical breakdown had been passed. In a liquid, this effect is not seen. Partial transmission occurs with each pulse of the mode-locked train. The percentage of energy transmission is reduced once optical breakdown occurs, but total energy transmission does not drop below the level of energy transmitted by pulses below the threshold for optical breakdown.[14, 17, 18] Figure 3–2 illustrates the difference in shielding of a mode-locked pulse train by gases and liquids, and Figures 3–3 and 3–4 show the similar plasma shielding and breakdown thresholds by three ophthalmic Nd-YAG lasers in model ocular media.

The lack of enhanced shielding by a mode-locked pulse train in liquid, as opposed to gas, indicates that the plasma in a liquid collapses in less than the 5 nsec between pulses. This reduction in plasma lifetime in liquids compared with gases is reasonable, because a liquid can be regarded as a very dense, or pressurized, gas in which the free electrons are kept in close proximity to the positive ions. In the absence of energy input between picosecond-long pulses, the electron avalanche ceases, and the plasma collapses before the next pulse arrives. The possibility of sustaining the plasma between pulses through partial mode-locking is theoretically interesting but remains unproved.[15]

In addition to absorption, the plasma scatters light by processes known as Brillouin scattering and stimulated Brillouin scattering. In Brillouin scattering, the light is scattered by thermally excited acoustic waves and shifted in a frequency equal to the frequency of the phonons characteristic of the material. In stimulated Brillouin scattering, which occurs at higher irradiances, the laser

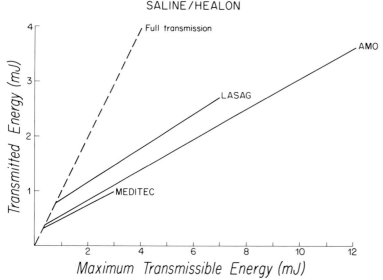

SALINE/HEALON

FIGURE 3–3

Transmission of energy by three ophthalmic Nd-YAG lasers focused in 0.9 per cent saline solution and in 1 per cent sodium hyaluronate. The curves for American Medical Optics (AMO) and Meditec have a statistically significant lower breakdown threshold than is found for the LASAG laser. (Reproduced from Steinert RF, Puliafito CA, Trokel S. Plasma formation and shielding by three ophthalmic Nd-YAG lasers. Am J Ophthalmol 96:427–34, 1983. With permission from Ophthalmic Publishing Co.)

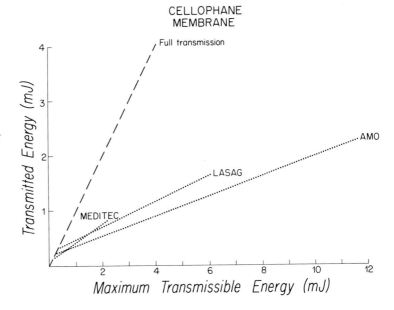

FIGURE 3–4

Transmission of energy by three ophthalmic Nd-YAG lasers focused on a cellophane membrane in 0.9 per cent saline solution. There was no statistically significant difference between the curves. (Reproduced from Steinert RF, Puliafito CA, Trokel S. Plasma formation and shielding by three ophthalmic Nd-YAG lasers. Am J Ophthalmol 96:427–34, 1983. With permission from Ophthalmic Publishing Co.)

light itself creates the acoustic wave that scatters it.[19] Stimulated Brillouin scattering is one of the mechanisms of laser material damage reviewed later in this chapter.

MECHANISMS OF DAMAGE IN CLINICAL THERAPEUTIC APPLICATIONS

Many mechanisms of damage have been described, depending on the target material, be it gas, liquid, or solid. Biologic tissues are more complex and variable than simple model targets, and so the clinical mechanisms of damage described are extrapolated from studies of the simpler targets.

Thermal Mechanisms. The microplasma temperature reaches 15,000°C focally.[20] Vaporization and melting of liquids and solids occur in a small volume near the focal point.[21, 22] In biologic systems, *thermal denaturation* of protein and nucleic acids is calculated to be confined to a radius of 0.1 mm for a 1-mJ pulse.[23] Therefore, although high local temperatures occur briefly, total heat energy is low, and clinical photocoagulation is not important.

Pressure Waves. Several mechanisms may combine to generate pressure waves radiating from the zone of optical breakdown.[24–29] Foremost among these is the rapid *plasma expansion* that begins as a hypersonic (shock) wave.[24–26] A plasma-generated shock wave is shown in Figure 3–5. A second weaker source of hypersonic and sonic (acoustic) waves is stimulated Brillouin scattering, in which the laser light generates the pressure wave that scatters it.[19, 30] The focal heating can lead to a *phase change* (vaporization and melting) and *thermal expansion*, both of which generate acoustic waves.[27–29] The electric field of the laser light if sufficiently strong will deform a target through *electrostriction* (the mechanism that leads to simple Brillouin scattering[19]) and through *radiation pressure* caused by momentum transfer from photons to atoms during inverse bremsstrahlung.[10]

Estimates of the contributions of these various mechanisms are given in Table 3–1. The complexity of biologic systems and the varying experimental[24, 26, 31, 32] and theoretical[30, 32] derivations make these figures approximate at best, but they are useful for assessing relative contributions. For example, the electrostrictive stress from a 50-nsec pulse with energy density of 1 J/cm² is

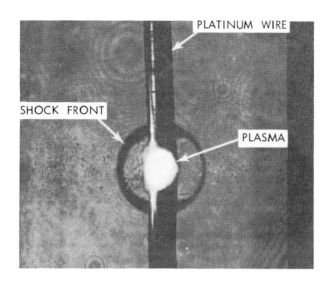

FIGURE 3–5

Shock wave in water. The shock wave is generated by a single laser pulse focused on platinum wire. The photographic delay was 70 nsec. The laser beam moved from left to right. (Reproduced from Bell CE, Landt JA. Laser-induced high pressure shock waves in water. Appl Phys Lett 10:46–8, 1967. With permission from the American Institute of Physics)

calculated at only 0.02 atm but may be as high as 80 atm for a 2 J/cm² 25 to 30 psec pulse (although the accuracy of this calculation is subject to some doubt).[32]

The shock wave begins immediately with plasma formation and expands at a hypersonic velocity of 4 km/sec. The wave front propagation falls to sonic velocity (1.5 km/sec in water) within 200 μ. The acoustic transient lasts 50 nsec at a location 300 μ from the focal point. The pressure falls from a maximum of 1000 atm to 100 atm within a distance of 1 mm.[31]

The shock wave is followed by cavitation or vapor bubble formation. Cavitation begins within 50 to 150 nsec after breakdown in water, expands rapidly for the first 20 μsec, reaches a maximum size of about 0.6 mm at 300 μsec, and collapses within 300 to 650 μsec.[25, 26] Cavity propagation velocity is approximately 20 m/sec at a point 300 μ from the breakdown.[33] Cavitation is too rapid to be visible and should be distinguished from bubble formation. Persistent bubbles probably consist of hydrogen and oxygen gas.[20]

Because impurities lower the threshold for optical breakdown, multiple shock waves can be generated along the laser beam path as impurities are encountered.[24, 25, 34]

Figure 3–6 combines current data on plasma shock wave and cavitation propagation to present a hypothetical model. The plasma shock wave propagates outward on a nanosecond time scale, dropping rapidly in amplitude and slowly widening (Fig. 3–6A). The cavitation process begins later with expansion and collapse on a microsecond time scale (Fig. 3–6B).

TABLE 3–1. ESTIMATED CONTRIBUTIONS TO PRESSURE WAVE AFTER OPTICAL BREAKDOWN

Mechanism	Maximum Pressure (Atmospheres)
Plasma formation	1000–2000
Stimulated Brillouin scattering	50–100
Phase change (vaporization)	100
Thermal expansion	100
Electrostriction	0.01–100
Radiation pressure	0.01

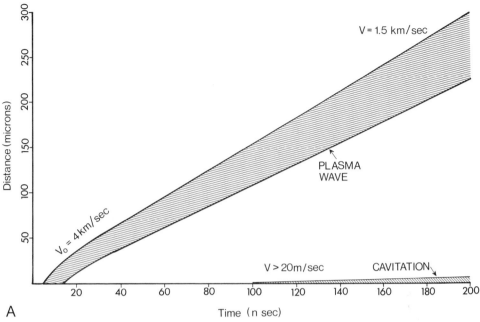

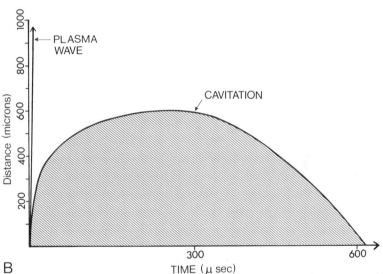

FIGURE 3–6

Conceptualization of plasma shock wave and cavitation after optical breakdown in liquid. *(A)* The plasma pressure-induced wave begins at hypersonic speed ($V_0 = 4$ km/sec) and rapidly slows to sonic velocity (1.5 km/sec) as it propagates outwardly. *(B)* Cavitation begins around 100 nsec at an initial velocity exceeding 20 m/sec. The bubble reaches a maximum size after about 300 μsec and collapses within about 600 μsec.[20, 21, 24, 25, 31, 33]

The size of the damage zone depends on (1) the level of irradiance and total energy input (up to a saturation level[35]); (2) the duration for which the plasma is sustained; and (3) the mechanical properties of the target tissue (density, mass, tensile strength, and elasticity).[15] Figure 3–7 summarizes the therapeutically relevant mechanisms of damage.

A scanning electron micrograph of an experimental Nd-YAG laser capsulotomy shown in Figure 3–8 illustrates the effects of these mechanisms of tissue damage.[36] The anterior capsule is sharply opened, and the underlying anterior cortex is disrupted.

Spark Emission. The visible spark represents the release of energy as photons when electrons recombine with ions (bremsstrahlung). The emission has a blackbody-like spectrum, including the visible, ultraviolet, and in some materials the near ("soft") X-ray wavelengths. The amount of ultraviolet emission is believed to be greater for picosecond-long than for nanosecond-

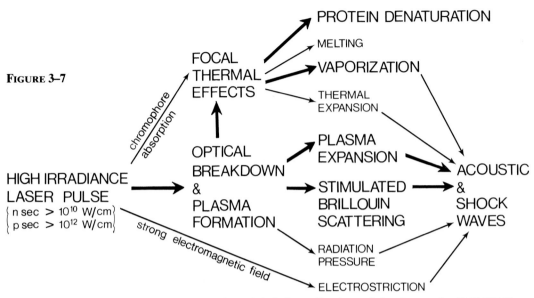

FIGURE 3–7

Clinically relevant mechanisms of damage in ophthalmic applications of the short-pulsed Nd-YAG laser. Dominant mechanisms are highlighted by heavy arrows and boldface type.

long induced sparks, but even in the case of picosecond-long pulses calculations indicate that toxicity to corneal epithelium would occur only for breakdown closer than 1.5 mm.[37] The spark is a useful marker of the zone of optical breakdown. The spark light emission itself is thus not a mechanism of therapeutic damage and has only limited potential toxicity.

Electromagnetic Field Stress. Limited evidence suggests that the electromagnetic field of a short laser pulse could exceed the electrical stress limit of

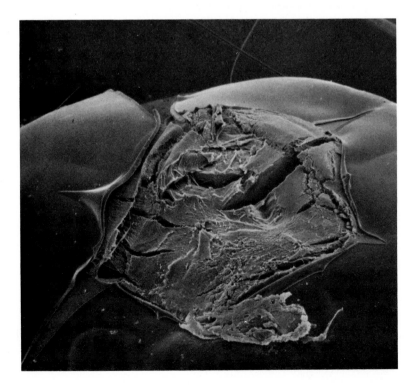

FIGURE 3–8

Scanning electron micrograph recorded one hour after Nd-YAG anterior capsulotomy in a rabbit eye. Note the sharply demarcated anterior capsule border and partial destruction of anterior cortex. Original magnification 20×. (Reproduced from Puliafito CA, Steinert RF. Laser surgery of the lens: Experimental studies. Ophthalmology 90:1007–12, 1983. With permission from *Ophthalmology*)

the membranes of some cells and organelles. On this basis the retinal photo-receptors theoretically may be vulnerable to picosecond-long pulses focused closer than 8.5 mm and to nanosecond-long pulses focused closer than 4.4 mm from the retina.[37] These values are only calculated, and direct experimental confirmation has not been made. If such damage occurred in the outer segments of the retina, however, it might be undetectable by the usual clinical techniques of ophthalmoscopy and fluorescein angiography. Localized electrophysiologic abnormality and histopathologically visible changes should occur. Further investigations of this mechanism of potential damage are needed.

Electromagnetic field stress is the mechanism for electrostriction and radiation pressure, which are two of the minor sources of pressure waves.

OPTICAL PROPERTIES NEAR THE FOCAL POINT

The high irradiance and plasma growth lead to focal point behavior not seen with lower-power linear optical phenomena.

Self-Focusing and Self-Trapping. Self-focusing can be induced by very high-power laser beams. The electrostriction of the electric field increases the index of refraction of the medium through which the laser beam passes.[38, 39] Self-focusing of the beam and continued propagation as a thin "filament" (self-trapping), illustrated in Figure 3–9, are seen only with the very high irradiance of picosecond-long pulses from mode-locked lasers[40, 41] and not from nanosecond-long Q-switched pulses. In ophthalmic lasers, the relatively strong final beam convergence should minimize or prevent the tendency for self-focusing.

PLASMA GROWTH AND PRELOADING

Self-focusing and self-trapping are unrelated to the other causes of breakdown occurring outside the expected focal spot. These causes include (1) impurities in the media, with lower breakdown thresholds,[24, 25, 34] (2) use of suprathreshold energy levels such that breakdown occurs before the smallest focal spot is reached (preloading), and (3) "hot spots" of increased irradiance caused by aberrations in the focusing lens and optical elements in the eye.[42–44] Suprathreshold pulses affect both the location at which breakdown first occurs and the direction of growth of the plasma. Because the threshold for optical breakdown depends on irradiance (W/cm^2), suprathreshold power pulses achieve breakdown at a larger spot than do threshold pulses (Figure 3–10A and B), that is, at a location anterior to the expected focal point. In addition, the plasma tends to spread in the direction of the incoming light, as depicted in Figure 3–10C, in a multilobed configuration.[45, 46] The "growth" fills the angular cone defined by the converging laser beam. The anterior growth of the plasma may be understood as the absorption of incoming light by the plasma. Absorption and further growth of the plasma thus occur at the anterior boundary of

FIGURE 3–9

High electric field strength in picosecond-long pulses induces an increase in the refractive index of the medium and leads to self-focusing and self-trapping of the laser beam with multiple breakdown regions in the form of a filament (after Loertscher[49]).

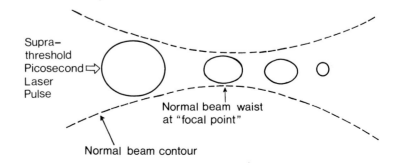

Supra-
threshold
Picosecond ⇨
Laser
Pulse

Normal beam waist
at "focal point"

Normal beam contour

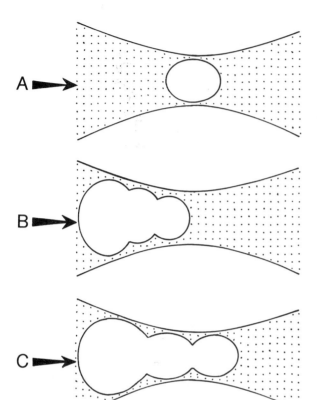

FIGURE 3–10
Growth of plasma anterior to the predicted focal point: *(A)* a threshold pulse with spherical breakdown at the beam waist; *(B)* a greatly suprathreshold pulse attains breakdown threshold anterior to the minimal spot size; *(C)* a moderately suprathreshold pulse extends toward the laser source in a multilobed configuration.

plasma first encountered by the incoming light. Posterior extension of breakdown is not seen in the absence of self-focusing and filamentation unless the irradiance is so great that suprathreshold levels of laser energy pass through the plasma, which is improbable. Several technical mechanisms have been proposed to fully explain observed plasma growth patterns.[47]

Studies by John D. Hunkeler, using a Q-switched ophthalmic Nd-YAG laser, confirm that increasing the energy level above the breakdown threshold causes the breakdown region to elongate along the beam path in a multilobed configuration. Figure 3–11 shows this phenomenon in a saline test chamber.

DAMAGE TO INTRAOCULAR LENSES

The frequent clinical application of ophthamic Nd-YAG lasers for posterior capsulotomy in the presence of adjacent intraocular lenses makes an understanding of the mechanism of damage in transparent solids particularly relevant.

Damage takes the form of melted voids, microcracks, and large pulverized regions. The breakdown in glass and polymethylmethacrylate (PMMA) caused by a Q-switched nanosecond-long pulse can have a filamentary character[48] that is suggestive of self-focusing and self-trapping not seen in liquids with Q-switched pulses. Damage caused by picosecond-long pulses is also filamentary in form.[40] The Q-switched pulse damage threshold for PMMA is about 10^8 W/cm^2 and that for glass is about 10^{10} W/cm^2. These thresholds are consistent with the recent observation that glass intraocular lenses (IOLs) may be more resistant to marking at low power levels, although damage, once it occurs, is more extensive.[49]

Cumulative effects have been found. The damage threshold of PMMA has

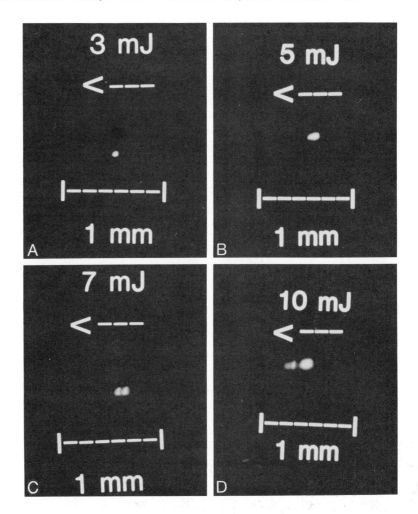

FIGURE 3–11

Photographs of spark formation from optical breakdown by a Q-switched ophthalmic Nd-YAG laser focused into a physiologic saline bath. The laser beam passes from right to left. *(A)* A threshold pulse shows a nearly round spark; *(B)* increase in energy causes area of breakdown to elongate; *(C)* multilobed breakdown is seen at double the threshold energy; *(D)* at triple the threshold energy, a greatly elongated multilobed breakdown region is seen that is approximately ten times longer than the breakdown zone seen at threshold *(A)*. (Courtesy of John D. Hunkeler)

been observed to drop by a factor of three after four or five successive laser shots.[50] Thus use of bursts of laser shots for posterior capsulotomy may lead to greater marking of an IOL than does the use of single shots.

The issue of whether the breakdown threshold changes with laser wavelength has become pertinent with the advocacy by some of the superiority of the Q-switched erbium-yttrium-lanthanum-fluoride (Er-YLF) laser over the Nd-YAG laser for posterior capsulotomy. The Er-YLF laser is designed to produce a pulse at 1228 nm. The proponents of the use of this laser contend that the threshold for capsulotomy is lower and the threshold for IOL damage is higher at this wavelength than with Q-switched Nd-YAG pulses at 1064 nm.[51] Quantitative studies of PMMA damage at these wavelengths are lacking. One study of breakdown thresholds in ruby and sapphire indicates a modest increase of the breakdown threshold as wavelength increases.[52]

The damage threshold is lower at the surface of a solid than in the interior,[53–55] particularly in the presence of surface irregularities.[56, 57] Clinically this effect can lead to preferential breakdown at the posterior surface of an IOL when the laser is aimed at an adjacent posterior capsule.

The mechanisms of damage in PMMA and glass are complex. Typical saucerlike cracks oriented 45 degrees to the axis of the laser beam that are seen in PMMA are best explained by hypersonic shock waves.[49] Structural inhomogeneities such as microcracks may serve as starting points for breakdown. Heating and vaporization near the focal point of the laser can be expected to cause melting and cracking,[21] but not all damage can be explained by this model alone. Thermal effects are believed to be less important than the shock wave generated by stimulated Brillouin scattering [49] and impact ionization.[52]

IOL manufacturing techniques and materials that minimize inhomogeneities, impurities, and inclusions and that result in a highly polished surface therefore should reduce the tendency for IOL damage during posterior capsulotomy. The surgeon should avoid surface damage through careful handling and insertion techniques. In performing laser posterior capsulotomy in the presence of a lens with scratches or deposits, such as in fibrin or inflammatory cells, the surgeon should anticipate an increased tendency for IOL marking by the laser. Clinical strategies for reducing IOL marking are discussed in Chapter 7.

REFERENCES

1. Frank-Kamenetskii DA. Plasma: The Fourth State of Matter. New York: Plenum Press, 1972, pp 1–39, 134–5.
2. Maker PD, Terhune RW, Savage CM. *In* Grivet P, Bloembergen N (eds.). Quantum Electronics, Proceedings of the Third International Congress. New York: Columbia University Press, 1964, p 1559.
3. Nelson P, Veyrie P, Berry M, Durand Y: Experimental and theoretical studies of air breakdown by intense pulse of light. Phys Lett 13:226–8, 1964.
4. Fradin DW, Bloembergen N, Letellier JP: Dependence of laser-induced breakdown field strength on pulse duration. Appl Phys Lett 22:635–7, 1973.
5. Ready JF. Effects of High-Power Laser Radiation. New York: Academic Press, 1971, pp 133–43.
6. Ibid., pp 137–40, 215–7.
7. Milam D. Can a model which describes gas breakdown also describe laser damage to the bulk and surfaces of solid dielectrics? *In* Glass AJ, Guenther AH (eds.). Laser Induced Damage in Optical Materials (7th Symposium, 1975). Washington: United States Government Printing Office, 1976, pp 350–5.
8. Bass M, Barrett HH. Avalanche breakdown and the probabilistic nature of laser-induced damage. IEEE J Quantum Electron QE-8:338–43, 1972.
9. Fradin DW, Yablonovitch E, Bass M. Confirmation of an electron avalanche causing laser-induced bulk damage at 1.06 microns. Appl Opt 12:700–9, 1973.
10. Ready JF. op cit., pp 261–2.
11. Smith DC, Haught AF. Energy-loss processes in optical-frequency gas breakdown. Phys Rev Lett 16:1085–8, 1966.
12. Mitsuk VE, Savoskin VI, Chernikov VA. Breakdown at optical frequencies in the presence of diffusion losses. JETP Lett 4:88–90, 1966.
13. Smith DC, Tomlinson RG. Effect of mode beating in laser produced gas breakdown. Appl Phys Lett 11:73–5, 1967.
14. Steinert RF, Puliafito CA, Trokel S. Plasma formation and shielding by three ophthalmic Nd-YAG lasers. Am J Ophthalmol 96:427–34, 1983.
15. Mainster MA, Sliney DH, Belcher CD, Buzney SM. Laser photodisruptors: Damage mechanisms, instrument design, and safety. Ophthalmol 90:973–91, 1983.
16. Puliafito CA, Steinert RF. Laser surgery of the lens: Experimental studies. Ophthalmol 90:1007–12, 1983.
17. Steinert RF, Puliafito CA, Kittrell C. Plasma shielding by Q-switched and mode-locked Nd-YAG lasers. Ophthalmol 90:1003–16, 1983.
18. Orlov RY, Skidan IB, Telegin LS. Investigations of breakdown produced in dielectrics by ultrashort laser pulses. Sov Phys JETP 34:418–21, 1972.
19. Ready JF. op cit., pp 279–83.
20. Barnes PA, Rieckhoff KE. Laser-induced underwater sparks. Appl Phys Lett 13:282–4, 1968.
21. Ponomarenko BF, Samoilov VI, Ulyakov PI. Polarization-optical investigation of the failure of transparent dielectrics by laser radiation. Sov Phys JETP 27:415–9, 1968.
22. Ready JF. op cit., p 301.
23. Hu C-L, Barnes FS. The thermal-chemical damage in biological material under laser irradiation. IEEE Trans on Bio-Med Eng BME 17:220–9, 1970.
24. Bell CE, Landt JA. Laser-induced high pressure shock waves in water. Appl Phys Lett 10:46–8, 1967.
25. Felix MP, Ellis AT. Laser-induced liquid breakdown—a step-by-step account. Appl Phys Lett 19:484–6, 1971.
26. Lauterborn W. High-speed photography of laser-induced breakdown in liquids. Appl Phys Lett 21:27–9, 1972.

27. Hu C-L. Spherical model of an acoustic wave generated by rapid laser heating in a liquid. J Acoust Soc Am 46:728–36, 1969.
28. Cleary SF, Hamrick PE. Laser-induced acoustic transients in the mammalian eye. J Acoust Soc Am 46:1037–44, 1969.
29. Carome EF, Clark NA, Moeller CE. Generation of acoustic signals in liquids by ruby laser-induced thermal stress transients. Appl Phys Lett 4:95–7, 1964.
30. Brewer RJ, Rieckhoff KE. Stimulated Brillouin scattering in liquids. Phys Rev Lett 13:334–6, 1964.
31. Van der Zypen E, Fankhauser F, Bebie H, Marshall J. Changes in the ultrastructure of the iris after irradiation with intense light. Adv Ophthalmol 39:59–180, 1979.
32. Cleary SF. Laser pulses and the generation of acoustic transients in biological material. *In* Wolbarsht ML. Laser Applications in Medicine and Biology, Vol. 3. New York: Plenum Publishing Corporation, 1977, pp 175–219.
33. Fujimoto J, Steinert RF, Puliafito CA. Unpublished data.
34. Carome EF, Carreira EM, Prochaska CJ. Photographic studies of laser-induced pressure impulses in liquids. Appl Phys Lett 11: 64–6, 1967.
35. Sigrist MW, Kneubuhl FK. Pressure saturation of laser-induced acoustic waves in liquids. Appl Phys Lett 34:353–4, 1979.
36. Puliafito CA, Steinert RF. Laser surgery of the lens: Experimental studies. Ophthalmol 90:1007–12, 1983.
37. Taboada J. Interaction of short laser pulses with ocular tissues. *In* Trokel S. YAG Laser Ophthalmic Microsurgery. Norwalk, CT: Appleton-Century-Crofts, 1983, pp 15–38.
38. Smith WL, Liu P, Bloembergen N. Superbroadening in H_2O and D_2O by self-focused picosecond pulses from a YAlG:Nd laser. Phys Rev A 15:2396–403, 1977.
39. Chiao RY, Garmire E, Townes CH. Self-trapping of optical beams. Phys Rev Lett 13:479–82, 1964.
40. Belozerov SA, Zverev GM, Naumov VS, Pashkov VA. Breakdown of transparent dielectrics by radiation from mode-locked lasers. Sov Phys JETP 35:158–60, 1972.
41. Anthes JP, Bass M. Direct observation of the dynamics of picosecond-pulse optical breakdown. Appl Phys Lett 31:412–4, 1977.
42. Evans LR, Morgan CG. Intensity distribution of focused laser beams in bio-medical studies. Phys Med Biol 14:205–12, 1969.
43. Aaron JM, Ireland CLM, Morgan CG. Aberration effects in the interaction of focused laser beams with matter. J Phys [D]: Appl Phys 7:1907–17, 1974.
44. Bryant GW, Schmid A. Contribution of spherical aberrations to the vestige structure induced by laser damage. J Opt Soc Am 71:764–70, 1981.
45. Young M, Hercher M, Wu C-Y. Some characteristics of laser-induced air sparks. J Appl Phys 37:4938–40, 1966.
46. Alcock AJ, DeMichelis C, Hamal K, Tozer BA. H-1-A mode-locked laser as a light source for schlieren photography. IEEE J Quantum Electron QE-4:593–7, 1968.
47. Ready JF. op cit., pp 266–9.
48. Ashkinadze BM, Vladimirov VI, Likhachev VA, Ryvkin SM, Salmanov VM, Yaroshetskii ID. Breakdown in dielectrics caused by intense laser radiation. Sov Phys JETP 23:788–97, 1966.
49. Loertscher H. Laser-induced breakdown for ophthalmic applications. *In* Trokel S (ed.). YAG Laser Ophthalmic Microsurgery. Norwalk, CT: Appleton-Century-Crofts, 1983, pp 39–66.
50. Likhachev VA, Ryvkin SM, Salmanov VM, Yaroshetskii ID. Fatigue in the optical damage of transparent dielectrics. Sov Phys-Solid State 8:2754–5, 1967.
51. Horn GD, Johnston M III, Arnell LE, Van Duyne RP. A new "cool" lens capsulotomy laser. Am Intraocul Implant Soc J 8:337–42, 1982.
52. Zverev GM, Mikhailova TN, Pashkov VA, Solov'eva NM. Mechanisms of destruction of ruby and leucosapphire crystals by powerful laser radiation. Sov Phys JETP 26:1053–7, 1968.
53. Hack H, Neuroth N. Resistance of optical and colored glasses to 3 nsec laser pulses. Appl Opt 21:3239–48, 1982.
54. Milam D. Laser-induced damage at 1064 nm, 125 psec. Appl Opt 16:1204–13, 1977.
55. Ready JF. op cit., p 289.
56. Bloembergen N. Role of cracks, pores, and absorbing inclusions on laser induced damage threshold at surfaces of transparent dielectrics. Appl Opt 12:661–4, 1973.
57. Austin RR, Michaud R, Guenther AH, Putnam J. Effects of structure, composition, and stress on the laser damage threshold of homogenous and inhomogenous single films and multilayers. Appl Opt 12:665–76, 1973.

4

LASER-TISSUE INTERACTIONS AND THE EYE

The electromagnetic spectrum is composed of radiant energy that ranges from very short cosmic waves (10^{-5} nm) to the longest radio waves (1000 meters) (Fig. 4–1). Laser output currently ranges from the far ultraviolet to the far infrared portions of the spectrum (Fig. 4–2). A correspondingly wide range of effects (both adverse and therapeutic) may be expected following the interaction of laser radiation with ocular structures. Large gaps in our knowledge regarding these interactions remain. Our understanding of the specific molecular events that follow laser irradiation of living systems is fragmentary. In fact, to date the development of ophthalmic lasers has been largely empirical, employing those wavelengths, pulse widths, and irradiances that were readily available. As new laser sources are developed and as laser biology advances, one goal is the creation of selective laser therapeutic approaches, in which desirable biochemical, cellular, and tissue effects are enhanced and unwanted damage is confined. Notwithstanding our current limited understanding of the fundamentals of laser photobiology, the eye is the organ in which laser effects have been most carefully studied, and a large volume of experimental and clinical information has been gathered. The goal of this chapter is to summarize the present knowledge of laser-tissue interactions in the eye.

BASIC CONSIDERATIONS

Radiation can be considered energy in transit. Electromagnetic radiation that can be propagated in a vacuum as well as in matter has features of both waves and particles. In the wave model, light is composed of rapidly alternating electric and magnetic fields oriented transversely to the direction of wave travel and perpendicular to each other. Some properties of light, such as refraction or scattering, can be explained on a macroscopic level by wave theory.

Photobiologic events, however, can be understood best by considering electromagnetic radiation to be composed of particles, that is, *photons*. Photons are discrete "packets" of light energy. The photon is the fundamental unit of exchange in all photobiologic transactions. As described in Chapter 3, the

36

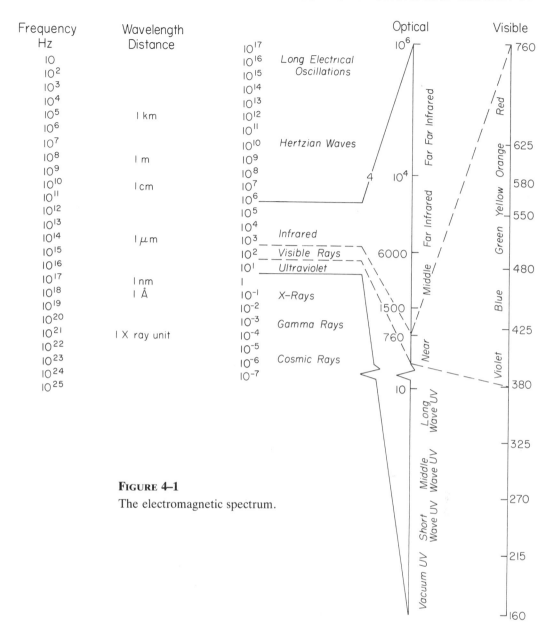

FIGURE 4–1

The electromagnetic spectrum.

energy of each photon is directly proportional to its frequency and can be described by the equation $E = h\nu = \dfrac{hc}{\lambda}$, where ν is the frequency in $\sec^{-1}$, λ is the wavelength, c is the speed of light in vacuum, and h is Planck's constant $(6.624 \times 10^{-34}$ joules $\cdot$ sec). That is, the longer the wavelength, the lower are the frequency and the photon energy. A 200-nm photon is five times more energetic than a 1000-nm photon.

The first law of photochemistry (Grotthus-Draper) states that photon absorption is absolutely necessary for a reaction to occur.[1] Photon absorption is the first event in the initiation of all photobiologic events. Absorption is a very specific event, determined by photon energy and the electronic configuration of the biomolecule. Figure 4–3 summarizes the events that occur after photon absorption. Photon absorption may result in ionization, bond breaking,

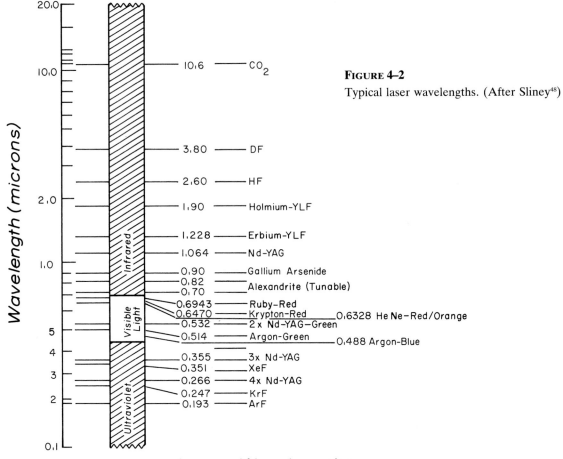

FIGURE 4–2
Typical laser wavelengths. (After Sliney[48])

Laser Wavelengths

electron excitation, or vibrational excitation. Absorption of highly energetic X-ray photons can produce ionization (that is, removal of electrons from the absorbing molecule). Ultraviolet photons may have sufficient energy to directly break chemical bonds. Absorption of photons in the ultraviolet and visible regions may produce electron excitation—that is, one of the absorbing atom's electrons goes into an unoccupied level with higher energy. When the excited atom returns to the ground state, energy may be emitted as light (phospho-

FIGURE 4–3

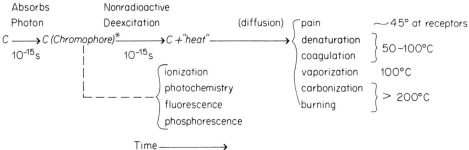

General sequence of physical events occurring when photon absorption, excitation, and dissipation of the absorbed energy cause radiant heating of matter. *C* represents a light-absorbing biomolecule or chromophore. (Courtesy of R. Rox Anderson)

rescence, fluorescence, spontaneous emission, or stimulated emission) or as heat. Absorption of lower-energy infrared photons produces an increase in the vibrational and rotational states of molecules, which is realized as an increase in temperature.

Chromophores are those molecules or portions of molecules responsible for the absorption of light energy. Chromophores are ubiquitous in living systems. Amino acids and nucleic acids absorb strongly in the ultraviolet range. As a result, cells and tissues absorb radiation strongly between 200 nm and 315 nm. Fewer biomolecules act as chromophores in the 400- to 1000-nm region (visible to near infrared range).[2] Among these are the important ocular chromophores of melanin, hemoglobin, and xanthophyll. In the infrared region, virtually all biomolecules have specific and strong vibrational absorption bands. Water, which is a prime constituent of all tissue, is an important chromophore that has a number of absorption bands in the midinfrared region.[3, 4]

The characteristics of both the target tissue and the laser source determine the biologic consequences of laser irradiation. Relevant tissue characteristics include spectral transmission and absorbance, scattering, distribution of chromophores within the target tissue, thermal conductivity and diffusivity, and convection. Important laser characteristics are wavelength, pulse duration, irradiance, and radiant energy. Laser effects in tissue can be classified roughly into three groups: thermal, photochemical, and ionizing. Included in the third group are optical breakdown and plasma formation, which are the two events that are central to photodisruption. These processes have been discussed in Chapter 3.

THERMAL EFFECTS: TRANSMISSION, ABSORPTION, AND SCATTERING

Until the advent of ophthalmic photodisruption, most therapeutic laser-tissue interactions relied on the production of thermal effects in the target tissue. As already discussed, the radiant energy of photons can be absorbed by biomolecules and converted to heat. Heat is transferred beyond the immediate target site by passive thermal diffusion or by convection (as by blood flow). The temperature rise produced by laser irradiation is a function of time, laser energy, laser wavelength, and the optical and thermal properties of the absorber.[5] A moderate increase in temperature under 100°C is associated with breakage of hydrogen bonds and van der Waal's forces, which stabilize the conformation of biologic macromolecules, such as proteins.[6, 7] The result of these conformational changes may be loss of biologic activity (enzyme inactivation) or structural integrity (alterations in cell membranes). This process, thermal denaturation, is complex and leads to cell death, hemostasis, and coagulation as well as a host reparative response (such as inflammation).

The ocular medium transmits light between wavelengths of 380 and 1400 nm (Fig. 4–4). In principle, light throughout this interval may be used to treat intraocular structures by delivery through the pupil. At wavelengths shorter than 380 nm the ultraviolet absorbing properties of the lens and cornea limit retinal exposure. At wavelengths longer than 1400 nm water absorption sharply limits transmission. Because laser light is monochromatic, highly collimated, and intense and because the eye is an optically open system, laser irradiation is well suited to produce thermal denaturation of intraocular tissue targets. This process is the basis for retinal photocoagulation.[8–10] The process of chorioretinal heating by laser irradiation has not only been modeled, but direct measurements have been reported of the temperature rise in rabbit and monkey retinas after argon laser irradiation.[10–13]

The ocular chromophores in the visible region are melanin (present in the

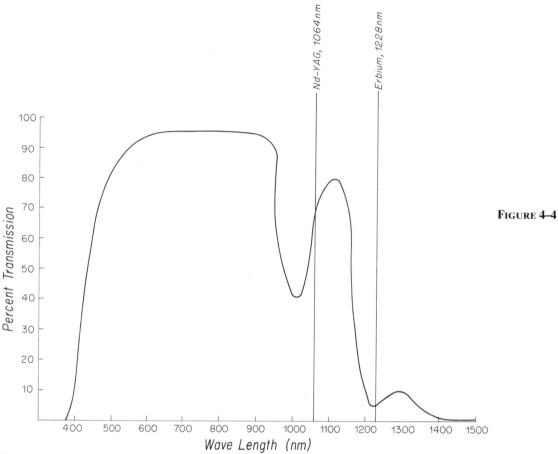

PERCENT TRANSMISSION THROUGH OCULAR MEDIA

FIGURE 4–4

Spectral transmission curve of ocular media. (After Geeraets and Berry, 1968[49])

retinal pigment epithelium, iris pigment epithelium, uvea, and trabecular meshwork), hemoglobin (present in blood vessels), and xanthophyll (present in the inner and outer plexiform layers of the retina in the macula). Each has a characteristic absorption spectrum (Figs. 4–5 to 4–7). Argon blue-green (composed primarily of the 488- and 514.5-nm emission lines), argon monochromatic green (514.5-nm), and krypton red (647-nm) are commonly employed in ocular photocoagulation. Krypton yellow (568-nm) and continuous-wave and long-pulsed neodymium-YAG (1064-nm) sources have also been used for photocoagulation.

Scattering as well as absorption can be an important determinant of laser tissue effects. In the normal eye, the ocular media have low scattering coefficients across the visible and near infrared spectrum, in a manner consistent with the function of vision. The amount of scattering is related to the wavelength of the incident light as well as the size and refractive index of the scattering particles. Molecular scattering can be described by Rayleigh's theory, in which scattering of particles with a size that is smaller than one tenth the wavelength is inversely proportional to the fourth power of the wavelength ($1/\lambda^4$). That is, light of shorter wavelength is scattered more than light of longer wavelength. Compared with scattering of larger particles, molecular scattering is weak, isotropic, and polarized. For ultraviolet and short-wavelength (blue) visible radiation, Rayleigh scattering is more important than for longer wavelengths;

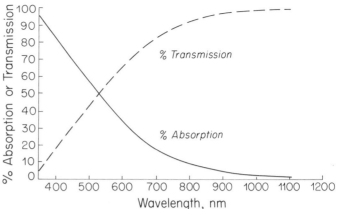

FIGURE 4–5

Absorption and transmission curves of the retinal pigment epithelium. (After Gabel, 1978[50])

however, scattering of larger particles, when present, generally dominates over molecular scattering. Turbidity of the ocular media (as in cataract or vitreous hemorrhage) is almost always primarily based on large-particle scattering.

So-called large-particle scattering is best described by Mie's scattering theory, which applies to particle sizes on the order of the wavelength and larger. Mie scattering is stronger and much more forward-directed than Rayleigh scattering. This characteristic, as described by Mie, is based on the interference of multiple Rayleigh scattering centers "within" each large particle. The intensity and forward-directedness of Mie scattering increases with particle size, with the limit for very large particles being equivalent to that set by the classic laws of refraction and reflection described by geometric optics. Turbid ocular media are caused by particle scattering in which there is relative disarray of particles or structures on the order of the wavelength or larger in size, with a refractive index differing from that of the media surrounding each particle. The wavelength-dependence of large particle scattering is much less than that of molecular scattering, but there is still an inverse relationship with wavelength. This type of scattering is therefore generally of greater pathologic importance.

FIGURE 4–6

Absorptivity spectrum of oxygenated hemoglobin. (After Welsch, et al., 1978[51])

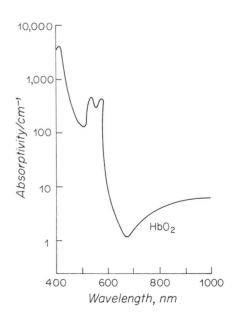

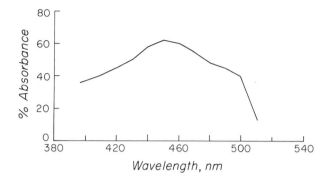

FIGURE 4–7
Absorption spectrum of xanthophyll. (After Gabel, 1978[50])

ARGON AND KRYPTON PHOTOCOAGULATION

The argon laser has proven efficacy in reducing the rate of severe visual loss when it is used for panretinal photocoagulation in eyes with proliferative diabetic retinopathy[14] and for photocoagulation of choroidal neovascular membranes 200 to 2500 microns from the center of the foveal avascular zone.[15] The target ocular chromophores for producing the desired therapeutic effects in retinal photocoagulation are melanin in the retinal pigment epithelium and hemoglobin in the retinal and choroidal vessels. The retinal pigment epithelium is the major site of absorption of both argon and krypton radiation.[16, 17] Despite the favorable spectral matching of argon laser light with hemoglobin, there is good experimental evidence that the primary therapeutic effect of the argon laser in closing choroidal vessels, for instance, is related to energy absorption in the melanin of the pigment epithelium. Because 647-nm light is not absorbed well by hemoglobin, the krypton red laser relies completely on absorption by melanin in the retinal pigment epithelium and choroid, with thermal transfer to vessels, to achieve obliteration of choroidal neovascularization.[18, 19]

In argon laser trabeculoplasty, the target chromophores are collagen and melanin in the trabecular meshwork. One mechanism proposed for trabeculoplasty is laser-induced shrinkage of meshwork collagen with secondary opening of meshwork lamellae.[20]

NEODYMIUM-YAG LASER PHOTOCOAGULATION

Neodymium-YAG lasers can be designed so that the temporal configuration of their output is continuous-wave or long-pulsed (200 microseconds to 20 msec). At these lower peak powers, thermal tissue effects predominate. A continuous-wave Nd-YAG laser that was used for experimental photocoagulation produced histologic lesions that were similar in appearance to those produced by lasers using krypton red.[21] Light of 1064 nm has low absorption in melanin compared with argon green or krypton red and penetrates much deeper. Fankhauser has reported the use of 10-msec Nd-YAG pulses for retinal photocoagulation.[22] 1064-nm radiation has a relatively low absorbance in hemoglobin and relies on absorption in surrounding pigmented tissue or scattering inside the blood vessels to produce coagulation. The deep penetration of 1064-nm radiation may have some undesirable consequences. Fankhauser and Van der Zypen reported that in experimental animals Nd-YAG retinal photocoagulation with 10-msec pulses stimulated fibroblast proliferation that penetrated Bruch's membrane and invaded the retina.[23] Fankhauser also reported a small series of cases in which he performed laser trabeculoplasty with 10-msec Nd-YAG pulses.[22] The efficacy of this technique or its equivalence or superiority to argon laser trabeculoplasty is unknown.

VAPORIZATION AND ACOUSTIC EFFECTS

Vaporization of tissue water (boiling) occurs when temperatures higher than 100°C are achieved. This liquid-to-gas phase change is associated with a dramatic volume expansion. For example, the production of steam at atmospheric pressure causes a 1700-fold volume expansion. Tissue damage occurs because of the formation and collapse of vapor cavities within tissue as well as by propagation of acoustic waves that cause mechanical damage.[24, 25]

The target chromophore for the carbon dioxide laser in biomedical applications is tissue water. Because the absorption coefficient of water is extremely high (950 cm^{-1}) at this laser's far infrared output of 10.6 μ, 99 per cent of the laser's output is absorbed within a distance of 100 μ, and the peak temperature rise generated occurs within the first 50 μ of tissue.[26] This strong tissue absorbance and the carbon dioxide laser's capability of producing high tissue irradiance make it an excellent laser for surface ablation of tissue. Heat diffusion away from the area of tissue ablation coagulates adjacent vessels and provides hemostasis. The carbon dioxide laser has been used in ocular surgery to penetrate the sclera in filtering surgery for glaucoma[27] and for transection of experimental vitreous membranes and liquefaction of vitreous gel.[28, 29] Because the carbon dioxide laser's infrared output cannot be transmitted via conventional glass or quartz fiber, an articulated arm delivery system or thallium bromoiodide (KRS-5) fibers have been employed.[30]

Laser pulse width is an important determinant of the tissue response to any given laser irradiation.[31, 32] For a given exposure energy, as pulse width decreases the peak temperature achieved in the target increases, since there is less time for thermal diffusion to adjacent structures. For sufficiently short pulses, adiabatic heating occurs; that is, there is virtually no loss of energy by diffusion from the target during the exposure. In this situation, the temperature of the target increases linearly with input energy, and if the incident energy is high enough vaporization occurs. Such an event can be observed clinically as gas bubble formation during retinal photocoagulation with a pulsed laser source.[33] As noted previously, laser-induced vaporization is accompanied by the formation of acoustic transients (pressure waves) that can produce mechanical damage to tissue. If the pulse is short enough, even if the total absorbed energy is less than the threshold for vaporization, acoustic transients can be produced without vaporization. The radiant exposure necessary for the production of acoustic transients is less than that necessary for vaporization.[34] Indirect evidence for the importance of such acoustic transients in producing damage in living systems comes from the observation that the energy necessary for producing threshold retinal lesions (in the absence of optical breakdown) is lowest for picosecond-long pulses and lower for nanosecond-long pulses than for millisecond or continuous-wave exposures.[35]

The fact that decreasing laser exposure pulse width decreases thermal diffusion (and therefore thermal injury) to tissue sites adjacent to the laser-irradiated area may be clinically useful in the future. Anderson and Parrish have proposed a general strategy (selective photothermolysis) in which a short intense burst of laser energy is used to heat the site of the absorbing chromophore to a temperature at which denaturation but not vaporization occurs.[36] The target cools by thermal diffusion to adjacent tissue sites that do not reach the critical temperature for thermal denaturation and damage.

PHOTOCHEMICAL DAMAGE MECHANISM

Sliney has recently summarized the features of laser-induced photochemical retinal injury. It is associated with exposure durations of longer than ten seconds; the visible appearance of the injury is delayed (latency); the effect is limited to short wavelengths (higher photon energies); and reciprocity of irradiance and exposure duration is observed.[37] The mammalian retina has been shown to be quite sensitive to photochemical damage produced by blue and near-ultraviolet light.[38] Photoreceptor as well as retinal pigment epithelial injury have been documented histologically. The chromophores for the initiation of such damage have not been definitively established.

Therapeutic use of laser-induced photochemical damage mechanisms in ophthalmology to date has been limited. One example is photoradiation therapy (PRT) employing hematoporphyrin derivative (HPD).[39] Hematoporphyrin is a photosensitizing agent that preferentially localizes in a variety of tumors. HPD converts absorbed light energy into a highly reactive species of oxygen, *singlet oxygen,* which produces oxidative damage that may result in cell death. Although HPD has a high absorption peak at 402 nm (blue light), 624-nm light (red) is employed for activation of HPD, since this wavelength has a higher degree of tissue penetration. This monochromatic light can be generated using a xenon light source or dye laser system. PRT has been employed in the treatment of a small number of patients with choroidal melanoma and retinoblastoma, and its efficacy is still under investigation.[40]

The development of excimer lasers that can efficiently generate high-power ultraviolet light has prompted the use of short-pulsed ultraviolet radiation for tissue ablation. Excimer laser light at 193 nm and 248 nm has been used to ablate corneal tissue.[41] It has been hypothesized that the excimer laser can produce spatially confined tissue ablation by direct photochemical bond breaking. The target chromophore for the initiation of effects would appear to be tissue protein and nucleic acids. Light microscopic examination of corneal tissue adjacent to the zone of ablation showed no evidence of coagulation necrosis, and this finding has been suggested as evidence that photochemical rather than thermal effects predominate in this application. However, the absence of thermal denaturation in adjacent tissue may also be related to the short pulse width of the laser irradiation (typically 10 nsec), which would limit thermal diffusion to surrounding structures. The relative importance of thermal and photochemical damage mechanisms in ultraviolet tissue ablation is not known. Moreover, concerns about the mutagenic and carcinogenic effects of ultraviolet light must be addressed.

PROTECTION OF THE RETINA IN PHOTODISRUPTION

Intense light that reaches the retina may cause chorioretinal damage related in a complex way to species, retinal pigmentation, site exposed, wavelength, pulse duration, spot size, total power and energy, irradiance and energy density of each exposure, total number of pulses, and rate of pulse delivery.

The irradiance necessary for a threshold injury increases with longer wavelengths for both short and long pulses.[42–44] In general, a shorter pulse has a lower damage threshold. For focused 1064-nm pulses of comparable spot size, a 25- to 35-psec pulse induces threshold-visible damage at 13 microjoules, compared with 68 microjoules for a 15-nsec Q-switched pulse, and the difference may be even larger.[45] For both long and short pulses, total energy and power to form a threshold lesion increase as retinal spot size increases, but the irradiance and energy density decrease as retinal spot size increases.[43, 46] With larger retinal images, cooling by choroidal blood flow may be slower in the center of the lesion. As a result, temperature elevation at the lesion center may be prolonged, with a resultant lower injury threshold. For Q-switched Nd-YAG pulses focused on the retina, repeated pulses at 10 Hertz (Hz) lower the threshold for retinal injury. This effect is not seen, however, for a large retinal spot size.[43] A thermal model has been proposed for the data on larger spot size.[35]

Therapeutic applications of the Nd-YAG laser employ energies many times in excess of the reported retinal damage thresholds. Therefore, it is necessary to consider how the retina is protected during pulsed YAG laser surgery. For a given laser with fixed wavelength and pulse duration, retinal protection is afforded by beam divergence and by the "shield" effect of plasma formation, which is discussed in Chapter 3. Beam divergence is defined as the angle formed by the cone of light converging upon and then diverging from the focal point of the delivery system. The "border" of the laser beam is variably defined as the $1/e$ or $1/e^2$ points or the solid angle (see pp. 16, 58). Commercial ophthalmic Nd-YAG lasers generally broaden the laser beam with an inverse Galilean telescope and then use a moderately large-diameter high-power final focusing lens to reach the desired combination of beam cone angle, minimal focal spot, and comfortable working distance.

Experimental studies have shown that retinal injury in a rabbit eye occurs during Nd-YAG laser capsulotomy if beam divergence does not reduce the energy density at the retina below the damage threshold.[47] Gaasterland's early clinical studies with his Q-switched ruby laser photodisruptor illustrated this point well. Using a cone angle of 7 degrees at the $1/e^2$ points of the beam and with the necessity of relatively high pulse energies, he noted retinal injury in six of nine patients treated in the anterior segment with this system. The typical appearance of such a lesion one hour and six months after treatment is illustrated in Figure 4–8. If the best experimental data for large retinal spot size exposures are used, a Q-switched Nd-YAG laser performing a capsulotomy 19 mm from the retina should reach the threshold for retinal injury only when the laser energy delivered to the cornea is 96 mJ. This is approximately 20 times the usual clinical maximal energy requirement for capsulotomy. For a 5-mJ pulse, beam divergence lowers irradiance below the retinal injury threshold at a distance of 4.3 mm from the focal point.

Figure 4–9 depicts the logarithmic relationship of the cone angle necessary to reduce retinal exposure to various energy density levels. If first order optics

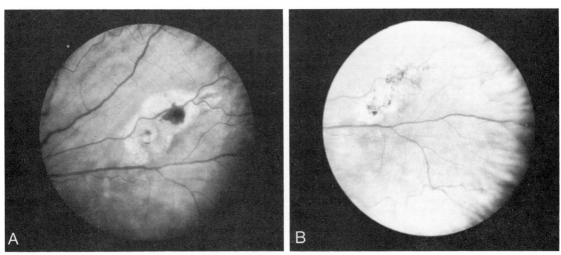

FIGURE 4–8   *(A)* Retinal injury following Q-switched ruby laser capsulotomy. This fundus photograph, taken one half hour after treatment, shows an area of retinal edema and retinal hemorrhage in the nasal retina. *(B)* Appearance of the same lesion six months after treatment. Note the hyperpigmented scar. (Courtesy of Douglas E. Gaasterland)

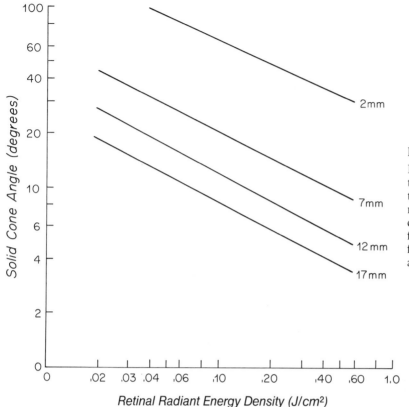

FIGURE 4–9

Logarithmic relationship of the solid cone angle necessary to achieve various retinal radiant energy density damage thresholds, calculated for a 5-mJ pulse, plotted at focal points located 2, 7, 12, and 17 mm from the retina.

are assumed and energy absorption by the ocular media is ignored, lines can be drawn to represent the relationship of cone angle to retinal radiant energy for a 5-mJ pulse. To maintain retinal exposure at a constant level, the necessary cone angle increases exponentially as the laser focal point approaches the retina.

If the threshold for retinal injury is in fact 0.40 J/cm^2 (rhesus monkey 900-μ spot),[43] a solid cone angle of 5 degrees should be adequate to just avoid retinal injury during posterior capsulotomy at 5 mJ. Therefore, Q-switched capsulotomy at 1 to 2 mJ with a 16-degree cone angle should be well below the retinal threshold.

For work in the pupillary plane, adequate beam divergence is the most important factor in retinal protection. Plasma formation is an additional means of reducing the radiant energy reaching the retina. Plasma formation absorbs and scatters incident radiation and thereby reduces the transmission of radiant energy along the beam path.

Plasma shielding may play an important role in retinal protection when the YAG laser is used to cut deep vitreous membranes. However, the plasma shield absorbs radiant energy (photons) and not the pressure waves that are generated by plasma expansion. Even if the transmission of radiant energy is decreased below the threshold for retinal injury by the plasma shield, if the zone of optical breakdown is adjacent to the retinal surface the acoustic and shock waves generated by the laser spark can propagate into the retina and choroid and cause injury. At the threshold for plasma formation, however, or if breakdown does not occur for a suprathreshold pulse, during anterior segment applications the beam divergence alone protects against retinal injury.

REFERENCES

1. Longsworth JW. Photophysics, luminescence and photochemistry. *In* Regan JD, Parrish JA (eds.). The Science of Photomedicine. New York: Plenum Publishing Corporation, 1982, p 43.
2. Hillenkamp F. Interaction between laser radiation and biologic systems. *In* Hillenkamp F, Pratesi R, Sacchi CA. Lasers in Biology and Medicine. New York: Plenum Press, 1980, pp 37–68.
3. Sliney D, Wolbarst ML. Safety with Lasers and Other Optical Sources. New York: Plenum Press, 1980, p 145.
4. Lund DJ, Stuck BE, Beatrice ES. Biological Research in Support of Project *MILES*. Report No. 96. San Francisco: Letterman Army Institute of Research, 1981.
5. Birngruber R. Thermal modeling in biologic tissues. *In* Hillenkamp F, Pratesi R, Sacchi CA. Lasers in Biology and Medicine. New York: Plenum Press, 1980, pp 77–97.
6. Lapanje S. Physiochemical Aspects of Protein Denaturation. New York: John Wiley & Sons, 1978, pp 56–76, 193–205.
7. Joh M. A Physico-Chemical Approach to the Denaturation of Proteins. New York: Academic Press, 1965.
8. Cummins L, Nauenberg M. Thermal effects of laser radiation in biological tissue. Biophys J 42:99–102, 1983.
9. Mellerio J. The thermal nature of retinal laser photocoagulation. Exp Eye Res 5:242–8, 1966.
10. Mainster MA, White TJ, Tips JH, Wilson PW. Transient thermal behavior in biologic systems. J Math Biophys 32:303–14, 1970.
11. Mainster MA, White TJ, Tips JH, Wilson PW. Retinal temperature increases produced by intense light sources. J Opt Soc Am 60:264–70, 1970.
12. Mainster MA, White TJ, Allen RG. Spectral dependence of retinal damage produced by intense light sources. J Opt Soc Am 60:848–55, 1970.
13. Priebe LA, Cain CP, Welch AJ. Temperature rise required for production of minimal lesions in the *Macaca mulatta* retina. Am J Ophthalmol 79:405–13, 1975.
14. The Diabetic Retinopathy Study Research Group. Photocoagulation treatment of proliferative diabetic retinopathy: The second report of the Diabetic Retinopathy Study findings. Ophthalmology 85:82–105, 1978.
15. Macular Photocoagulation Study Group. Argon laser photocoagulation for senile macular degeneration: Results of a randomized clinical trial. Arch Ophthalmol 100:912–8, 1982.
16. Marshall J, Bird AC. A comparative histopathologic study of argon and krypton laser irradiations of the human retina. Br J Ophthalmol 63:657–68, 1979.
17. Editorial. Search for the ideal laser. Br J Ophthalmol 10:655–6, 1979.
18. Singerman LJ. Red krypton laser therapy of macular and retinal vascular diseases. Retina 2:15–28, 1982.
19. Yanuzzi L. Krypton red laser photocoagulation for subretinal neovascularization. Retina 2:29–46, 1982.
20. Thomas J. Laser trabeculoplasty. *In* Belcher CD, Thomas JV, Simmons R. Photocoagulation in Glaucoma and Anterior Segment Disease. Baltimore: Williams & Wilkins, 1984, p 64.
21. Peyman G, Conway M, House B. Transpupillary CW YAG laser coagulation. A comparison with argon green and krypton red lasers. Ophthalmology 90:992–1002, 1983.
22. Fankhauser F. The Q-switched laser: Principles and clinical results. *In* Trokel S (ed.). YAG Laser Ophthalmic Microsurgery. Norwalk, CT: Appleton-Century-Crofts, 1983, pp 128–31.
23. Van der Zypen E, Fankhauser F, Loertscher HP. Retinal and choroidal repair following low power argon and Nd-YAG laser irradiation. Doc Ophthalmol Pro Series 36, 1983.
24. Cleary SF. Laser Pulses and the Generation of Acoustic Transients in Biological Material. *In* Wolbarsht ML (ed.). Laser Applications in Medicine and Biology. Vol. 3. New York: Plenum Press, 1977, pp 175–219.
25. Cleary SF, Hamrick PE. Laser induced transients in the mammalian eye. J Acoust Soc Am 46:1037–44, 1969.
26. Mainster MA. Ophthalmic applications of infrared lasers: Thermal considerations. Invest Ophthalmol Vis Sci 18:414–20, 1979.
27. Beckman H, Fuller TA. Carbon dioxide laser scleral dissection and filtering procedure for glaucoma. Am J Ophthalmol 88:73–7, 1979.
28. Miller JB, Smith MR, Pincus F, Stockert M. Transvitreal carbon dioxide laser photocautery and vitrectomy. Ophthalmology 85:1195–1200, 1978.
29. Bridges TJ, Patel CKN, Strnad AR, Wood OR, Brewer ES, Karlin DB. Syneresis of vitreous by carbon dioxide. Science 219:1217–8, 1983.
30. Meyers SM, Bonner RF, Rodrigues MM, Ballintine EJ. Phototransection of vitreal membranes with the carbon dioxide laser in rabbits. Ophthalmology 90:563–8, 1983.
31. Van der Zypen E, Fankhauser F, Bebie H, Marshall J. Changes in the ultrastructure of the iris after irradiation with intense light. Adv Ophthalmol 39:59–180, 1979.
32. Wheeler CB. Introduction to lasers. J Roy Soc Med 76:813–5, 1983.
33. Kapany NS, Peppers NA, Zweng HC, Flocks M. Retinal photocoagulation by lasers. Nature 199:146–9, 1963.
34. Cleary, op. cit., pp 179–80.

35. Greiss GA, Blankenstein MF. Multiple pulse laser retina damage thresholds. Am Indust Hyg Assoc J 42:287–92, 1981.
36. Anderson RR, Parrish JA. Selective photothermolysis: Precise microsurgery by selective absorption of pulsed radiation. Science 200:524–7, 1983.
37. Sliney DH. Interaction mechanisms of laser radiation with ocular tissues. Presented at the Boulder Laser Damage Symposium, November 16, 1982.
38. Ham WT, Mueller HA, Ruffolo JJ, Guerry D, Guerry RK. Action spectrum for retinal injury from near ultraviolet radiation in the aphakic monkey. Am J Ophthalmol 93:299–306, 1982.
39. Dougherty TJ, Kaufman JE, Goldfarb A, Weishaupt KR, Boyle DG, Mittenar A. Photodisruption therapy in the treatment of malignant tumors. Cancer Res 38:2628, 1978.
40. L'Esperance FA. Ophthalmic lasers. 2nd ed. St. Louis: C.V. Mosby, 1983, pp 340–51.
41. Trokel SL, Srinivansan R, Braren B. Excimer laser surgery of the cornea. Am J Ophthalmol 96:710–5, 1983.
42. Gibbons WD, Allen RG. Retinal damage from suprathreshold Q-switch laser exposure. Health Phys 35:461–9, 1978.
43. Griess GA, Blankenstein MF, Williford GG. Ocular damage from multiple-pulse laser exposures. Health Phys 39:921–7, 1980.
44. Ham WT, Mueller HA, Sliney DH. Retinal sensitivity to damage from short wavelength light. Nature 260:153–5, 1976.
45. Ham WT, Mueller HA, Goldman AI, Newnam BE, Holland LM, Kubabara T: Ocular hazard from picosecond pulses of Nd-YAG laser radiation. Science 185:362–3, 1974.
46. Beatrice ES, Frisch GD. Retinal damage thresholds as a function of image diameter. Arch Environ Health 27:322–6, 1973.
47. Puliafito CA, Steinert RF. Laser surgery of the lens: Experimental studies. Ophthalmology 90:1007–12, 1983.
48. Sliney D. The optical spectrum: Laser and ultraviolet sources and standards. Presented at Lloyd's Conference on Radiation and Energy, December 9, 1983.
49. Geeraets WJ, Berry ER. Ocular spectral characteristics as related to hazards from lasers and other sources. Am J Ophthalmol 66:15–20, 1968.
50. Gabel VP, Birngruber R. Klinische Folerungen aus Xanthophylleinlagerung in der Netyhautnutte, Ber 76. Zus Dtsch Ophth Ges, 1968.
51. Welsch H, Birngruber R, Borgen KP, Gabel VP, Hillenkamp F. Spektrale Lichtabsoptin in Vollblut unter Beruchsichtigung der Streuung. Zus Dtsch Ophth Ges, 415, Bermann Verlag, Munich 1977.

5

INSTRUMENTATION

Various models of ophthalmic Nd-YAG lasers differ not only in basic laser parameters but, often more importantly, in delivery system design considerations that determine versatility, safety, convenience, and price. Within certain constraints, currently there is a large variation in system design. Furthermore, several of the earliest producers of ophthalmic Nd-YAG laser systems have made a number of ongoing evolutionary modifications as clinical experience grows. In this chapter specific commercial lasers are not compared; rather, the principles and application of laser system design for the ophthalmic Nd-YAG laser are explored. The reader then can use these design parameters as the basis for a rational comparison of specific models (see Table 5–1).

LASER SOURCE

The Laser Crystal and Wavelength. The most widely employed laser medium to produce optical breakdown is neodymium-yttrium-aluminum-garnet (Nd-YAG), with the major fundamental output at 1064 nm in the near-infrared range. Use of a weak emission line of Nd-YAG at 1300 nm has been proposed[1] but is not employed in any current commercial unit. Erbium-yttrium-lanthanum-fluoride (Er-YLF) is an alternative laser crystal with one of its emission lines at 1228 nm.[2] The use of longer wavelengths (within the range of high corneal transmission, which begins to drop significantly at wavelengths longer than 1300 nm) may theoretically reduce the threshold for optical breakdown, as explained on p. 33. Possible advantages of using longer wavelengths have been postulated.[1, 2] These advantages pertain to a decreased tendency for intraocular lens (IOL) marking and increased retinal safety in comparison with the use of 1064-nm wavelengths, as a result of increased absorption by the vitreous and decreased absorption by retinal and choroidal melanin (see Chapter 4). At 1064 nm delivered in current laser systems, however, IOL marking is a relatively minor problem (see discussion in Chapters 7 and 8), and retinal injury in anterior segment applications has not been demonstrated (see later discussion of beam divergence parameters; also see Chapter 4). Vitreous absorption of longer wavelengths may lead to undesirable vitreous heating and precludes treating posterior vitreous pathology. To establish any relative advantage of a given wavelength, extensive experimental studies with control of all of the other delivery system parameters are required.

TABLE 5–1. PULSED LASER PARAMETERS

Laser source	Controls
Crystal	Energy monitor
Wavelength (1064, 1228, 1300, 532 nm)	At laser cavity
Mode structure (TEM$_{00}$, other)	At end of system
Beam divergence (mrad)	Proper safety shutters
Pulsing	Convenience
Q-switch	Location
Mode-lock	Illumination
Dye change requirements	Protected location
Delay in pulse delivery?	Adjustments
Long-pulse? ("thermal")	Trigger
Duration	Hand/foot/both
Energy per pulse	"Heads-up" display
Energy range	Energy selection
	Continuously variable
"Burst" modes	Step intervals
Number of pulses per burst	Printout record?
Frequency (Hz)	He-Ne—YAG focus shift?
Pulse-to-pulse energy stability	Optical micrometer?
Cooling	Positioning
Air	Slit lamp controls
Internal recirculating water	Mechanical/motorized
Electrical requirements	Micromanipulator
Volts	Table adjustment
Amps	Vertical travel
Delivery systems	Wheelchair accommodation?
	Adjustable stool
Aiming beam	Motorized?
He-Ne	Photography
Single/dual/other	Video/35-mm/both
Stationary/rotating	***Costs***
Other	
Parfocal He-Ne and YAG?	Delivered price
Optical pathway	Taxes and duties
Assembly	Shipping
Fixed (above or below)	Warranties
Articulating arm	Laser head
Final pathway	System
In front of microscope and illumination	Service contract options
With illumination	Routine maintenance
Through slit lamp	Laser room
Slit lamp model	Wiring/lighting/plumbing
Beam conditioning optics	Warning lights
Cone angle (degrees)	Local building and safety codes
Solid angle	Manufacturer
$1/e$	Long-term stability and commitment
$1/e^2$	Reliability and service
Focal spot size (μ)	

Certain crystals can harmonically shift the wavelength of high-power laser output. For example, the harmonics of 1064 nm are 532 nm (green), 355 nm (near ultraviolet), and 256 (midultraviolet). There is no known clinical advantage to photodisruption at a shorter wavelength such as 532 nm. Unfortunately, the efficiency of these crystals depends on high peak power. Long-pulse ND-YAG emission because of lower peak power cannot be "frequency-doubled"* to 532 nm with adequate efficiency to be useful for green-light ophthalmic photocoagulation.

---

*Recall that $v = c/\lambda$, where λ is wavelength, v is frequency, and c is the speed of light. Doubling of the frequency halves the wavelength.

Mode Structure. As explained in Chapter 2, the fundamental mode (TEM_{00}) allows laser light to be focused to the smallest spot, and consequently optical breakdown is achieved with the least possible energy input. Most manufacturers therefore specify the TEM_{00} mode for optical breakdown applications. A low-order nonfundamental mode may be clinically acceptable if optical breakdown can be achieved at energy levels comparable with the threshold level with fundamental mode. The clinical benchmark is performing a posterior capsulotomy through a posterior chamber lens at 1 mJ of output energy delivered to the cornea.

Beam Divergence. The beam divergence as the light leaves the laser cavity also directly influences final spot size. The smaller the divergence, the smaller is the final focal spot. Beam divergence is measured in milliradians (mrad) and in ophthalmic Nd-YAG lasers typically ranges from 0.5 to 3 mrad.

Pulsing. As discussed in detail in Chapter 2, Q-switching results in a single pulse typically between 2 and 20 nsec in duration. Mode-locking gives a train of seven to ten 30-psec pulses each spaced 4 to 5 nsec apart. The pulse train therefore lasts 30 to 50 nsec. The mechanism of optical breakdown differs for Q-switched and mode-locked pulses, giving a more intermittent and "explosive" quality to a Q-switched pulse at threshold energy levels (see p. 25).

The most common Q-switch is an electro-optical device known as a Pockel's cell. These devices are widely used industrially and have high durability. Mode-locking in ophthalmic systems is currently obtained passively by use of a saturable dye. The dye periodically requires replacement, after a lifespan of one or many months, depending on use. Power output decreases as the dye ages, signaling the need for replacement. Systems with large reservoirs of recirculating dye and sealed replacement cartridges have made passive mode-locking dependable and dye-changing easy and infrequent. The mode-locked design should allow immediate delivery of a pulse train when the trigger is pressed. No perceptible delay should occur.

If the Q-switch is left open the laser output lengthens from between 200 microseconds to 10 to 20 msec (see Fig. 2–8), with a corresponding drop in peak power. In principle the longer pulse can be useful for photocoagulation. In Chapter 4 the tissue interaction of pulsed 1064-nm light is discussed. In fundamental mode lasers, maximal long-pulse energy is usually less than 500 mJ, which may be inadequate for many clinical applications. Precise and expensive mechanisms are necessary to shift back and forth from fundamental mode to multimode output. The multimode output includes more energy; up to 2 to 5 J of long-pulse energy may be obtained in multimode output.

Energy Range. Q-switched Nd-YAG multimode industrial lasers often emit pulses with energies of several joules. For ophthalmic applications, in fundamental mode or a low-order mode, maximal energy per pulse is usually between 10 to 20 mJ. Mode-locked Nd-YAG lasers have a maximum energy per pulse train of about 5 mJ.

Under ideal circumstances, most applications can be performed with less than 5 mJ. In the authors' experience the higher energies available with Q-switching are useful in cutting very dense material and in situations in which optical degradation of the quality of the beam occurs. Hazy media such as corneal edema or scarring, turbidity in the anterior chamber from pigment or blood, astigmatism caused by corneal scars, application through the peripheral cornea, and use of some gonioscopic lenses can all reduce the amount of energy reaching the focal spot and increase the minimal spot size. Increasing the pulse energy to 10 mJ or more can often achieve optical breakdown in the presence of these conditions.

"Burst" Modes. When the laser is set to fire a single Q-switched pulse or mode-locked train, most ophthalmic systems allow a firing rate between one and ten times per second (1 to 10 Hz). Both Q-switched and mode-locked systems can be designed to deliver a volley or "burst" of shots at a fixed rate. The operator selects the desired number of shots in the burst and then triggers the laser. Most commonly, from 2 to 5 to 9 shots per burst may be selected.

Current models commonly have burst repetition rates ranging from 10 to 100 Hz; several models have a repetition rate of 500 kiloHertz (kHz). These rates correspond to interpulse spacing of 0.1 second for 10 Hz, 20 msec for 50 Hz, 10 msec for 100 Hz, and 2 microseconds for 500 kHz. Fankhauser has recommended that burst duration not exceed 160 msec (a burst of 9 at 50 Hz) in order that the burst be completed before a patient can react and the target move, which would lead to inadvertent damage to adjacent structures.[3]

Use of a burst of shots instead of single shots has been advocated by some clinicians on the basis of subjectively "easier" tissue cutting, particularly with dense membranes or mobile tissue fragments. No clinical studies to substantiate this claim have been published. Studies were conducted in the authors' laboratory, using a 50-Hz burst mode Q-switched Nd-YAG laser to compare single shots with burst shots on model targets.[4] The results showed that both dense and mobile targets could be cut effectively by single shots or bursts. To achieve a given effect, the number of applications of the burst mode was moderately less than for single-shot applications. The total number of pulses was greater, however, for burst mode shots compared with single shots. This disparity became greater with increased burst pulse number. Therefore, total energy delivered to achieve a desired effect was greater with the burst mode than with single shots. The longer the burst, the greater is the relative inefficiency of the cutting. Mobile targets were observed to move in reaction to the burst within four pulses, making later pulses in the train less accurately focused. Because the burst mode delivers a large number of pulses rapidly, this mode achieved the desired end point somewhat more quickly than did single shots, despite the relative inefficiency of the burst mode. This probably accounts for the subjective impession of improved burst mode cutting reported by some clinicians. The inefficiency of bursts is probably due to anterior migration of the breakdown zone with successive pulses and posterior displacement of the target by the pressure waves of preceding pulses.

Different laser-tissue interaction may be present for burst modes at 500 kHz compared with 50 Hz, but no comparative studies have been reported.

Under any circumstance, burst mode posterior capsulotomy should be avoided in the presence of a posterior chamber lens because of the increased likelihood of IOL damage by repeated shots through the same area as well as the increased risk of damage caused by the patient's movement during the application of a burst. Deep vitreous use of the burst mode is also unwise, because of adjacent retina that may be injured through movement and because the retina may have a lower damage threshold with rapidly repeated shots.[5] No significant difference in plasma shielding occurs with burst mode applications compared with single shots.[6]

Pulse-to-Pulse Stability. When a Nd-YAG laser pulse is delivered to the patient, the operator relies on knowledge of the energy in the preceding pulse along with pulse-to-pulse stability in order to predict the energy of the next pulse to be emitted. This method differs from that for a continuous-wave laser like the argon laser, which has an ongoing steady output. The Bureau of Radiologic Health specifications require that individual shot energy vary no more than 10 per cent from the average energy. Pulse instability is one of the factors that has so far limited the use of cheaper, compact, military-designed Nd-YAG lasers for ophthalmic application.

Cooling. Cooling of the flash lamps and laser rod in pulsed opthalmic Nd-YAG lasers is by ambient air or internally recirculated cooled water. Use of external cold water cooling, which is common for argon lasers, is not necessary in current designs.

Electrical Requirements. Most current ophthalmic models operate on 110-V standard outlets. Amperage requirements may be up to 20 amps.

DELIVERY SYSTEMS

Aiming the Beam. A continuous-wave argon laser is attenuated between pulses by a filter that transmits a safe level of laser radiation to provide for aiming of the laser beam. A pulsed Nd-YAG system requires a separate aiming system because there is no emission between pulses and because of the invisible infrared wavelength. Most systems use a continuous-wave low-power helium-neon (He-Ne) laser to locate the focal point. The He-Ne laser emits a red beam at 632.8 nm with an irradiance level selected to be below the threshold for retinal injury. In principle, other light sources can also act as an aiming beam, but the focal qualities of laser light have made the He-Ne laser the most commonly employed source.

The He-Ne aiming beam is coaxial with the Nd-YAG pathway. The He-Ne beam may be transmitted as a single beam, in which case the focal point is the brightest and smallest spot. Alternatively, aperture or prism arrangements may be used to modify the He-Ne beam into an annulus (circle) pattern or into two or more separate beams. At the focal point all light converges into a single bright spot, but out of the plane the He-Ne beam appears as a circle in the case of the annulus or as two or more dots in the case of the multiple beams. Figure 5–1 illustrates this effect for a single beam, an annulus pattern, and a "dual" He-Ne beam. A study in the authors' laboratory revealed that the dual He-Ne beam provides the most exact focus.[7] Utilizing a micrometer stage, the "depth of focus" of the apparent focal point was measured. With the dual-

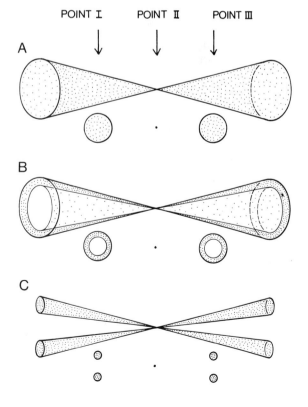

FIGURE 5–1

Schematic representation of three He-Ne aiming beam configurations and the pattern seen at three different points: Point I, anterior to the focal point; Point II, at the focal point; Point III, posterior to the focal point. Configuration *A* is a single "solid" beam; *B* represents an annulus or circle; *C* represents two beams or a "dual" He-Ne system.

beam system, the separation of the single spot into a dumbbell shape and then into two separate points was more readily discriminated by most observers than the enlargement and dimming of a single spot with the single beam or the formation of an annulus out of a single spot.

Not all dual-beam systems are expected to be equivalent. The smaller and sharper the two beams, the tighter will be the zone of convergence into a single spot.

Rotation of a dual-beam aiming system is designed to reveal whether part of the laser beam is being obstructed or cut off, such as at the edge of a gonioscopy mirror. This possible advantage must be weighed against the distraction of flashing reflections from every reflective surface. The annulus pattern should also reveal beam cutoff, as well as induced astigmatism, but unfortunately does not discriminate the focal point as well as does the stationary dual He-Ne beam.

One recently developed alternative aiming system uses an incandescent colored light angled from below relative to the slit lamp beam. At the focal point the colored light is centered in a gap in the white slit lamp beam. Anterior to the focus the colored light is below the gap; posterior to the focus the colored light is above the gap. The advantages and accuracy of such a system remain to be assessed.

Because of the difference in wavelength, the 1064-nm Nd-YAG beam comes into focus behind (posterior to) the 633-nm He-Ne beam, unless the manufacturer has specified an achromatic lens design for these two wavelengths.

Optical Pathway. Current fiberoptic technology does not satisfactorily transmit high peak power pulses. Thus all ophthalmic Nd-YAG laser systems bring the beam from the laser to the patient through air with fixed mirrors to direct the beam. The small Q-switched laser cavity has allowed most manufacturers to rigidly fix the laser to the slit lamp, from either above or below. This procedure avoids the use of a traditional articulating arm, which can go out of alignment more easily. Mode-locking requires a longer cavity and so such lasers are not rigidly fixed to the slit lamp. Current mode-locked models avoid an articulating arm, however, by use of a sliding subassembly under the slit lamp.

The choice of slit lamp partly determines the final beam pathway, as shown in Figure 5–2. Haag-Streit and Topcon style slit lamps usually bring the laser beam from below, either in front of or with the slit beam tower (Figs. 5–2A and B). With Zeiss, Nikon, and Rodenstock style slit lamps, the laser beam is commonly delivered through the final slit lamp objective lens, coming either from a laser mounted above the slit lamp or from below through a hollow support arm for the biomicroscope (Figs. 5–2C to E).

The final beam pathway involves certain design compromises. A single ideal configuration has not yet been marketed. If the laser beam exits in front of the slit lamp illumination, in a separate assembly, then a maximum independence and flexibility of the slit lamp microscope, the illumination, and the laser is obtained. In particular, the slit beam can be made truly coaxial with the laser beam, which is important for gonioscopic and vitreous applications. However, the assembly is exposed to potential damage, and the working space is reduced (Fig. 5–2A).

If the laser beam is brought in with the slit lamp illumination (Fig. 5–2B), the usual viewing position brings the laser beam obliquely through the cornea and IOL, which induce beam astigmatism and increase the chance of IOL marking. Ophthalmologists are accustomed to flexibility of slit illumination positioning and in most applications desire the laser beam to be coaxial with the optical pathway of the biomicroscope oculars.

Bringing the laser beam through the slit lamp body, either from above or below, produces the most externally protected design (Fig. 5–2 C to E). In the case of the Nikon FS-2 slit lamp, this may mean sacrificing variable magnification and photographic capability. In all cases, the usual slit lamp beam assembly blocks the laser beam if the slit beam is placed coaxially for gonioscopy or vitreous treatments. To avoid this problem, the slit beam tower may be lowered and angled upwardly, but true coaxial illumination is not present. Supplemental true coaxial illumination may still be necessary, especially for vitreous applications.

Beam-Conditioning Optics. The laser beam must be expanded by an inverse Galilean telescope and then brought into focus by a final converging lens. This optical assembly determines the cone angle of the laser beam and the final focal spot size.

As discussed in Chapter 4, the cone angle of the beam delivered to the patient is the major factor in retinal protection. The divergence of the beam after the focal point must reduce the irradiance at the retina below the threshold for retinal damage. The cone angle is usually specified in degrees. However, the definition of the boundary of the beam must be specified in comparing different systems. The three common definitions of the boundary are (1) the "solid angle" defined by the geometry of the laser aperture and the focal point, (2) the $1/e$ points containing 63 per cent of the energy, or (3) the $1/e^2$ points containing 86.5 per cent of the energy (refer to the definition of the $1/e$ and $1/e^2$ points on p. 16). Using these different definitions, true retinal irradiance can vary by a factor of nine.[8] These three definitions of cone angle are illustrated in Figure 5–3A.

Many current ophthalmic Nd-YAG lasers are specified to have a nominal solid cone angle of about 16 degrees. Practical design limitations of a slit lamp configuration limit the solid cone angle to about 20 degrees maximum. The larger the cone angle, the lower the irradiance is at a given distance in front of and behind the focal point. This is advantageous for reducing IOL marking during posterior capsulotomy. A larger angle of beam convergence allows a smaller focal spot, and thus lower energy to achieve optical breakdown, and reduces the tendency for anterior growth of the breakdown zone. Figure 5–3B illustrates the advantage of a 16-degree cone angle compared with a 9-degree cone angle with regard to the effect of "preloading," in which suprathreshold energy levels result in optical breakdown anterior to the nominal focal point. Breakdown occurs as soon as threshold irradiance (W/cm^2) has been achieved. Because area is a square function of radius, a small increase in cone angle causes a relatively large increase in the area being irradiated at a given distance anterior to the focal point.

The disadvantage of a large cone angle is the increased likelihood of "vignetting" or cutting off of a portion of the beam during gonioscopy or in work conducted through the pupil. Particularly for deep vitreous work, some manufacturers have advocated a smaller cone angle, which may be fixed or adjustable. Of course, a smaller cone angle increases retinal irradiance and limits the proximity to the lens and retina in which optical breakdown can safely be used. Figure 5–4 shows the aperture requirements for 9-degree and 16-degree solid beams to pass through the pupil and focus posteriorly. To focus 17 mm behind the pupil, a 16-degree solid-angle beam needs a pupil of 4.8 mm. If the clinician considers that this amount of pupillary dilation or more is necessary to visualize the posterior vitreous target with the contact lens, then there is reason to maintain the larger cone angle to better define the focal spot and reduce irradiance to adjacent structures (such as the retina and lens).

An ideal system may theoretically achieve a focal spot size of about 4 μ in diameter. Direct measurement of spot size in a high peak power laser is difficult and usually calculated indirectly. Therefore spot size specifications should be regarded as guidelines only.

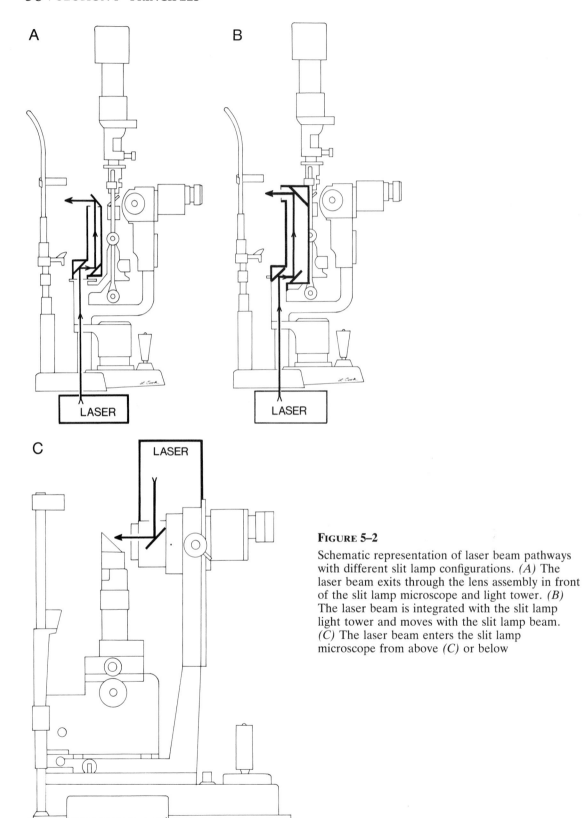

A

B

LASER

LASER

C

LASER

FIGURE 5–2

Schematic representation of laser beam pathways with different slit lamp configurations. *(A)* The laser beam exits through the lens assembly in front of the slit lamp microscope and light tower. *(B)* The laser beam is integrated with the slit lamp light tower and moves with the slit lamp beam. *(C)* The laser beam enters the slit lamp microscope from above *(C)* or below

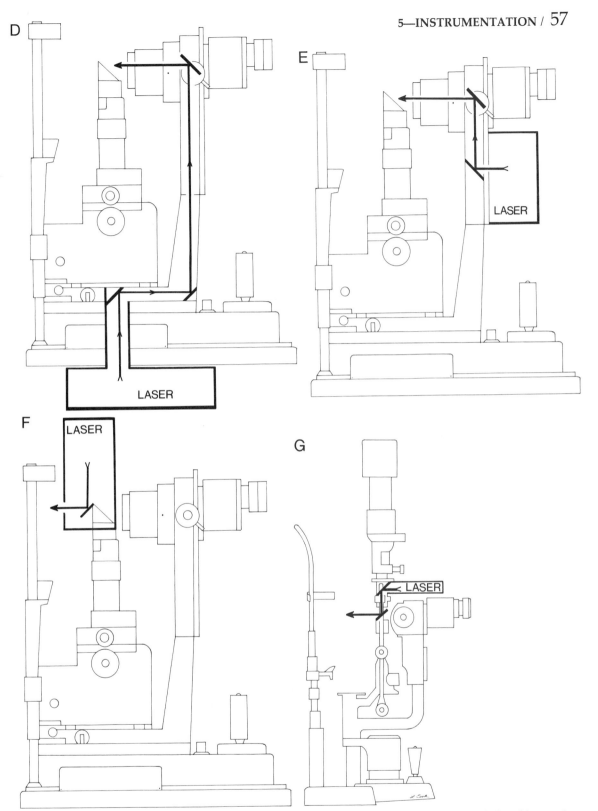

FIGURE 5–2
Continued

(D, E) and passes through the final objective lens of the microscope. If placed in a truly coaxial position, the slit lamp illumination arm will block the laser beam and therefore must be displaced laterally or inferiorly for designs *C, D,* and *E.* Small and lightweight lasers may be mounted directly on the slit lamp light towers *(F, G)* functionally equivalent to configuration *B.*

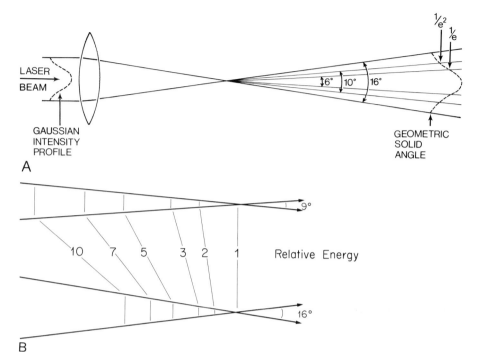

A

B

FIGURE 5–3 *(A)* The same optical beam can be labeled as 6, 10, or 16 degrees, depending on the definition of the boundary (after Sliney[8]). *(B)* Comparison of solid cone angles of 9 and 16 degrees with regard to the predicted anterior movement of optical breakdown. As input energy is increased (preloading) the threshold irradiance is achieved at larger areas before the focal point is reached. Because the area is a square of the radius, the anterior movement of the breakdown zone is much more pronounced for 9 degrees than for 16 degrees.

The overall performance of the optical system can be assessed best by the threshold for breakdown in distilled water (the invisible impurities in tap water enhance breakdown) or sterile physiologic saline solution. Air breakdown is unreliable because of the influence of humidity and particulate matter.

Controls. The Bureau of Radiologic Health standards require a key that limits operator access to the laser, an audible warning when the laser is armed, and shutters for the lasers (He-Ne and YAG), which are closed when the laser

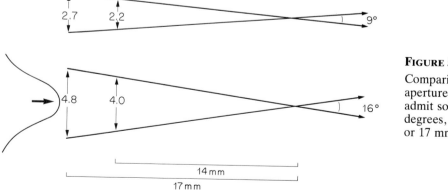

FIGURE 5–4

Comparison of pupillary aperture requirements to fully admit solid angles of 9 and 16 degrees, coming to a focus 14 or 17 mm behind the pupil.

is first activated and must be opened manually. The YAG laser should never be operated without the He-Ne shutter open.

To activate the YAG laser, a test sequence is necessary that includes a test shot into a closed shutter to monitor the energy output. Proper design should prevent change of the energy level, accidental or purposeful, when the shutter is open. The shutter should be closed and a test shot fired to determine the new energy setting.

Energy can be monitored at the laser cavity or near the end of the delivery system. The latter is preferable, since it more reliably monitors energy actually being delivered to the cornea.

While the physician is treating a patient, controls should be conveniently located in a position somewhat protected from accidental manipulation and illuminated for use in a darkened room. The trigger may be manipulated with a hand or foot control, or with the optional choice of either.

Several manufacturers have introduced a "heads-up" display that shows critical information, particularly the energy setting and the number of shots, in the slit lamp while the treatment is under way. This is a useful safety feature that helps to keep the physician aware of current treatment parameters.

Energy selection ideally can be varied in a continuous manner from zero to maximal range by a knob such as a volume control on a radio. Alternative systems are fixed or variable interval step adjustments and occasionally micro-computer programs.

Some laser models use a microprocessor to store treatment data and provide a printout as a permanent record at the end of the procedure.

As an approach to avoiding posterior chamber IOL marking during posterior capsulotomy, several models have a mechanized system to shift the He-Ne focus a fixed interval in front of the expected Nd-YAG breakdown zone. Of course, many optical and power variables influence the final location of the Nd-YAG breakdown, and the actual relationship of the YAG breakdown to the Ne-He focus may vary considerably.

An integrated optical micrometer that measures anteroposterior slit lamp travel with an accuracy of 10 μ has been introduced as another approach to avoiding posterior chamber IOL marking. The surgeon can focus on the capsule or IOL and then move a measured distance posteriorly. In vitreous work, the micrometer can be referenced to a known point (cornea, iris, lens, or retina) and then displaced to the target. The micrometer displays the focal point location and helps prevent inadvertent injury to adjacent ocular tissues. The micrometer reading should be displayed in a "heads-up" system and should be able to be zeroed at any desired reference point. A monitor to indicate proper stable head position is also mandatory.

Patient and Laser Positioning. Most systems move the laser beam in the target area with the slit lamp controls, whether manual or motorized. A micromanipulator that allows laser beam travel without moving the slit lamp may facilitate rapid treatment if the patient's position is steady.

Treatment is facilitated by the maintenance of a position that is comfortable to the patient. Up-and-down adjustment of the slit lamp support table is helpful. Ability to treat a patient in a wheelchair is occasionally very useful. A stable motorized adjustable stool is expensive but makes adjustment of the patient's orientation at the slit lamp easier.

Photographic Capability. Different models allow videotaping, 35-mm photography, or both. These are popular options for teaching and documentation.

Costs. Cost factors that should be considered in purchasing a unit include delivery price (including shipping, import duties, and taxes, if any), laser head warranty, system warranty, service contract options, routine maintenance

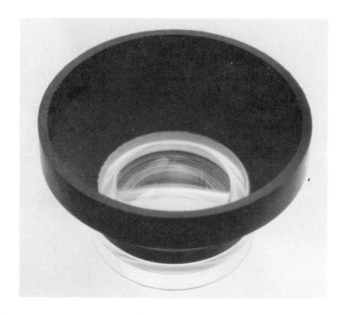

FIGURE 5–5

A YAG contact lens for posterior capsulotomy to stabilize the eye, prevent blinking, and maintain a good optical surface (Peyman 12-mm lens). (Photo courtesy of Ocular Instruments, Inc., Bellevue, WA)

including supplies (such as dye for mode-locked lasers), and the room for the laser. This last item involves wiring, lighting, sink, "laser-on" warning light, and local building and safety code requirements such as for door interlocks. A final major cost factor that can be only subjectively assessed is the stability and long-term commitment of the manufacturer and the reputation for reliability and service.

CONTACT LENSES

Contact lenses should not be mandatory for simple posterior capsulotomy. Beam convergence already should be present that is adequate for optical breakdown and retinal protection. A variety of lenses are useful for special

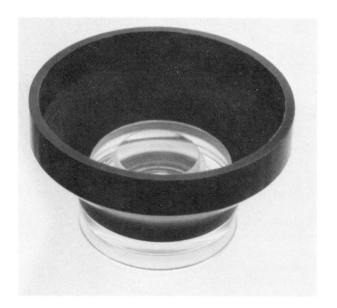

FIGURE 5–6

Central Abraham button lens for magnified posterior capsulotomy. (Photo courtesy of Ocular Instruments, Inc., Bellevue, WA)

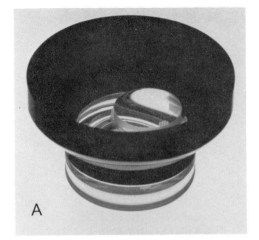

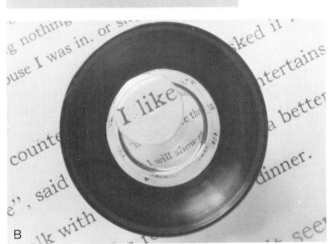

FIGURE 5–7

(A) Peripheral Abraham button lens for peripheral iridectomy. *(B)* Magnification provided by 66 diopter button. (Photos courtesy of Ocular Instruments, Inc., Bellevue, WA)

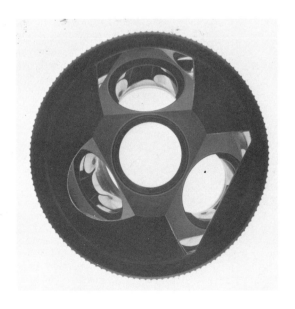

FIGURE 5–8

Conventional three-mirror Goldmann gonioscopy and fundus lens. (Photo courtesy of Ocular Instruments, Inc., Bellevue, WA)

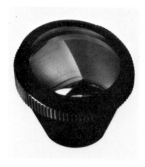

FIGURE 5–9

YAG design gonioscopy lens (Trokel lens). (Photo courtesy of Ocular Instruments, Inc., Bellevue, WA)

applications. If not supplied by the laser manufacturer, after-market lenses are available that are designed for YAG applications.

For posterior capsulotomy in the presence of a posterior chamber IOL, many physicians prefer a contact lens to stabilize ocular movements, eliminate blinking, and maintain the regular optical surface over the course of the treatment. One such lens is a compact lens with an anterior curvature similar to that of the usual cornea (8- to 12-mm radius of curvature) as shown in Figure 5–5. A central high plus power button lens may be added to increase beam convergence and magnify the surgeon's view, as in the Central Abraham lens with a 66 diopter button shown in Figure 5–6. Limitation of illumination and a smaller field of view through the button lens are drawbacks to this lens for some surgeons.

For peripheral iridectomy, a peripheral Abraham button lens (Fig. 5–7) is very useful because it improves visualization and control of the optical break-down process, especially in the critical situation of a YAG iridotomy over a noncataractous crystalline lens.

Gonioscopy treatments can be performed with standard mirror lenses as long as the laser is not misfocused so that it delivers a focused high irradiance pulse to the mirror that can damage the mirror (Fig. 5–8). Therefore, standard 3 mirror laser lenses usually can be employed, although lens manufacturers do not always approve of this use. A pupillary treatment must never be performed with this planosurface lens, since it eliminates the beam convergence of the cornea and makes retinal imaging possible.

Standard gonioscopic mirrors may be too small to accept the full beam cone of the laser, with consequent loss of power as a result of vignetting. Induced astigmatism can also be a major problem with conventional lenses. Special YAG gonioscopic lenses are being introduced to allow better angle visualization and treatment within a short working distance (Fig. 5–9).

For mid- and deep vitreous work, compact laser contact lenses with anterior curvature that ranges from flatter than the cornea to a planoanterior surface are available. Such lenses are similar in appearance to the lens shown in Figure 5–5 but have a flatter anterior surface.

REFERENCES

1. Peyman GA, Kraff M, Veherkoski E, Ressler N. Noninvasive capsulectomy using a new pulsed infrared laser. J Am Intraocul Implant Soc 8:239–46, 1982.
2. Horns GD, Johnston M III, Arnell LE, Van Duyne RP. A new "cool" lens capsulotomy laser. J Am Intraocul Implant Soc 8:337–42, 1982.
3. Fankhauser F. The Q-switched laser: Principles and clinical results. In Trokel SL (ed.). YAG Laser Ophthalmic Microsurgery. Norwalk, CT: Appleton-Century-Crofts, 1983, pp 101–46.

4. Steinert RF, Puliafito CA. Comparison of cutting efficiency by single shot and "burst mode" Nd-YAG lasers. In preparation.
5. Griess GA, Blankenstein MF, Williford GG. Ocular damage from multiple-pulse laser exposures. Health Phys 39:921–7, 1980.
6. Steinert RF, Puliafito CA, Trokel S. Plasma formation and shielding by three ophthalmic Nd-YAG lasers. Am J Ophthalmol 96:427–34, 1983.
7. Steinert RF, Belcher CD III, Wasson PJ, Puliafito CA. Aiming accuracy of different He-Ne beams for use with the ND-YAG laser. In preparation.
8. Sliney DH. YAG laser safety. *In* Trokel SL (ed.). YAG Laser Ophthalmic Microsurgery. Norwalk, CT: Appleton-Century-Crofts, 1983, pp 67–82.

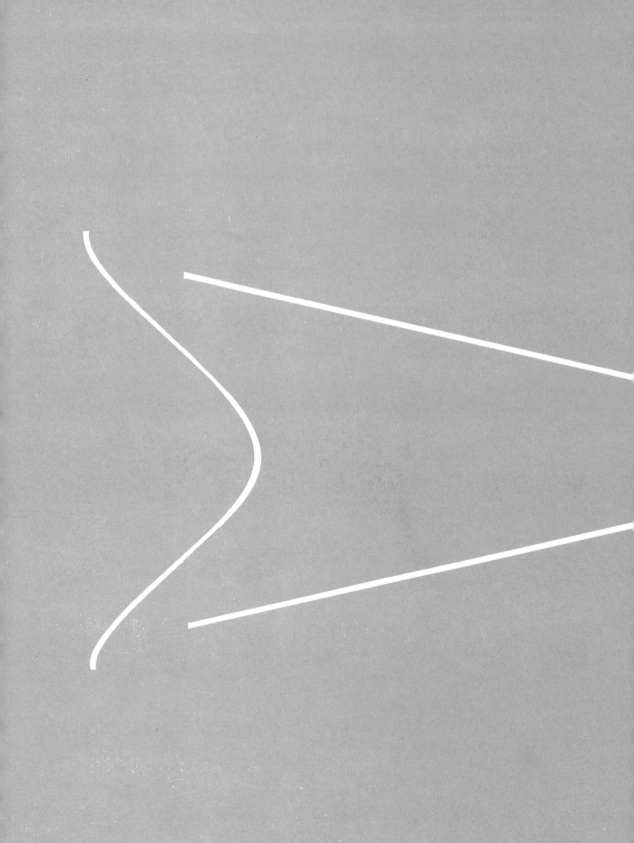

SECTION II

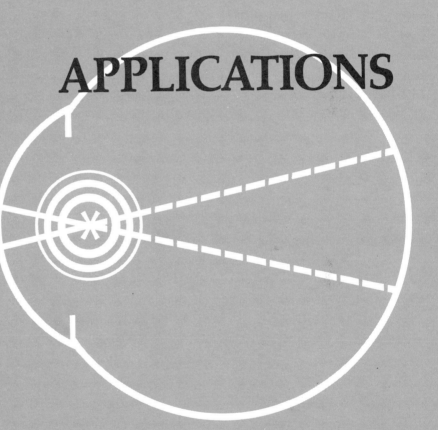

APPLICATIONS

6

PRINCIPLES OF CRITICAL FOCUS FOR CLINICAL APPLICATIONS

Successful clinical application of the Q-switched and mode-locked ophthalmic Nd-YAG laser requires achieving adequate irradiance for optical breakdown and having the optical breakdown occur at the intended target. To complete a pass, a quarterback must calculate the future location of a moving target, avoid defensemen, and include environmental factors such as wind, rain, and field conditions in determining the timing, arc of release, and strength of a pass. In ophthalmic microsurgery with the Nd-YAG laser, the surgeon is in an analogous position.

On a routine slit lamp examination, a patient may seem cooperative and to fixate steadily, but in the attempt to focus a 10-μ spot the surgeon suddenly becomes aware of previously unrecognized movements caused by heart beat, respiration, and patient anxiety and discomfort, as well as uncontrollable microsaccades during even optimal fixation. The surgeon must avoid nearby structures such as an intraocular lens (IOL), the iris, and the cornea. In addition, the optical properties of the cornea, anterior chamber, and IOL, plus a contact lens if used, interact with the energy of a laser pulse to influence the ultimate strength and location of optical breakdown. As the surgeon gains experience with clinical applications of the short-pulsed YAG laser, it becomes possible to rapidly make a calculation of these many interacting factors; many such calculations become virtually automatic. As is true for the quarterback, however, an appreciation of the principles of *critical focus* facilitates the acquisition of these skills. The clinical principles presented here are based on the physical principles developed in Section I, and references to Section I are given in subsequent discussions.

1. *Optical breakdown is a nonlinear process.* Breakdown occurs suddenly, when irradiance, or density of power, exceeds the threshold for optical breakdown (Chapter 3).

2. *Increasing energy input causes the breakdown zone to move anteriorly.* As converging light travels toward the focal point (or more precisely stated, the beam waist) of the lens system, the irradiance increases as the light power becomes increasingly condensed. Optical breakdown occurs as soon as the threshold power density is achieved; increasing the laser energy setting increases

the power so that the threshold power density is first achieved at a larger spot area, anterior to the smaller focal spot. The He-Ne focal spot remains stationary, while the apparent YAG focal spot moves toward the surgeon. Figure 3–10 illustrates this principle.

3. *Using the minimum necessary energy helps to keep the He-Ne and YAG lasers parfocal.* Suprathreshold energy increases laser-induced tissue damage by delivering more power, but anterior movement of the breakdown zone must be anticipated at the same time.

4. *The smaller the beam cone angle, the greater will be the anterior movement of a suprathreshold breakdown zone.* This differential shift of the breakdown zone with a 9-degree cone angle compared with a 16-degree cone angle is illustrated in Figure 5–3B.

5. *Suprathreshold energies result in an elongated breakdown region that extends anteriorly along the laser beam axis.* A suprathreshold pulse achieves breakdown anterior to the theoretical focal point (principle 2) and then continues to expand anteriorly along the beam axis (see Fig. 3–11). This process occurs primarily because the majority of the incoming laser energy is absorbed by the existing plasma, which in turn leads to further optical breakdown and plasma formation. This absorption and plasma growth occurs along the beam path toward the laser source.

6. *Predictable optical breakdown is degraded by media opacity.* Corneal scars or edema, or blood or pigment in the aqueous or on the intraocular lens, absorb and scatter light. Less laser power reaches the target, and the focal spot size becomes larger. Thus irradiance at the target decreases, and input energy must be increased to achieve the threshold irradiance for optical breakdown. Impurities in the media near the focal point may cause the breakdown to occur before the intended target is reached as a result of impurity-enhanced breakdown. This effect may be particularly prominent with Q-switched lasers (Chapter 3).

7. *Predictable optical breakdown is degraded by induced astigmatism.* Regular or irregular astigmatism may be induced by any of these mechanisms: (a) the normal peripheral cornea; (b) oblique passage through normal central cornea, an IOL, or a contact lens; and (c) corneal scars, surface irregularity, or astigmatism. Figure 6–1 illustrates each of these effects. An astigmatic beam cannot achieve as small a focal spot as can a normal beam and therefore requires increased energy input to achieve breakdown. Moreover, the break-

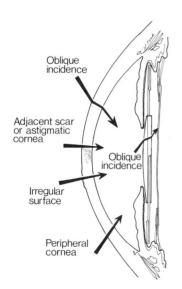

FIGURE 6–1

Sources of induced astigmatism in a laser beam passing through ocular structures. Induced astigmatism by a contact lens is not shown.

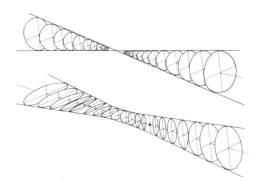

FIGURE 6–2

Astigmatism changes a well-defined beam waist *(top)* to
an elongated breakdown region *(bottom)*.

down zone is elongated by the induced conoid of Sturm (Fig. 6–2). In the case
of a posterior capsulotomy in the presence of a posterior chamber IOL, the
result can be an oblique IOL damage track through the body of the IOL.
Whenever possible, the laser pathway should be through central clear cornea,
perpendicular to the cornea and IOL. If the laser design delivers the laser
beam path coaxially with the slit lamp illumination (see p. 54), the illumination
should be central, and the eye should be viewed through the biomicroscope at
an angle through the peripheral cornea. For other designs in which the laser
beam path is coaxial with the biomicroscopic view, the usual clinical practice is
to position the microscope centrally with the slit lamp swung to the side. The
patient should be allowed to blink frequently to prevent epithelial drying, and
immediate prelaser pressure measurement and topical medications should be
avoided in order to maintain surface regularity. When marked corneal astigmatism or irregularity is present, use of a YAG contact lens reduces this
problem by shifting the air interface from the cornea to the optically superior
contact lens front surface.

8. *The threshold for optical breakdown is lower at optical interfaces than
in optically uniform media.* This physical property has several clinical consequences. (a) When threshold energy is employed for capsulotomy, breakdown
occurs if the laser is accurately focused on the capsule, but no breakdown is
seen if the laser is slightly misfocused in the aqueous or vitreous. The laser is
not malfunctioning; rather, the surgeon's focus is not adequately critical. (b)
If, in order to avoid posterior chamber IOL damage, breakdown in the anterior
vitreous is intended, then the energy setting must be higher than for achieving
threshold posterior capsule breakdown (see techniques in Chapter 7). (c) If a
posterior chamber IOL is in close proximity to the posterior capsule, the
breakdown may tend to "jump" toward the posterior IOL surface. If the laser
is focused slightly anterior to the posterior capsule, the capsule may remain
intact while the back of the IOL acquires a laser mark. Poor surface finish or
lens deposits increase this tendency. (d) The same effect occurs for applications
in the peripheral anterior chamber. In peripheral iridectomy or in cutting
vitreous strands adherent to a surgical wound the proximity of the cornea must
be remembered.

Inexact focus or suprathreshold energy levels may result in optical breakdown on the corneal endothelium. Figure 6–3 illustrates the lower breakdown
threshold at an optical interface.

9. *Use of a contact lens may enhance critical focus.* A YAG contact lens
that exactly duplicates the corneal surface does not alter beam convergence.
Critical focus may be enhanced, however, because of (a) an air interface that
is superior compared with the corneal tear film (see principle 7), (b) stabilization
of the eye, and (c) elimination of blinking and squeezing of the lids. A contact
lens that has a smaller anterior radius of curvature than the cornea acts as a
plus lens, increasing beam convergence, reducing focal spot size, and magnifying
the surgeon's view (Fig. 6–4).

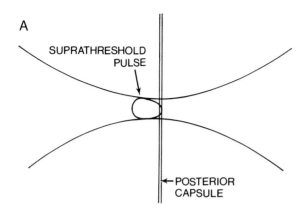

FIGURE 6–3

Effect of misfocusing anterior to the posterior capsule. *(A)* In aphakia, use of a suprathreshold beam uneventfully ruptures the posterior capsule, despite a tendency for optical breakdown to elongate anteriorly. *(B)* With a nearby pseudophakos, the breakdown threshold is lower at the optical interface of the IOL surface, and the breakdown occurs in a zone anterior to the aphakic case. The IOL is marked, and the capsule may even remain intact. Use of minimal energy and posterior focusing reduces this tendency for breakdown at an optical interface anterior to the beam waist.

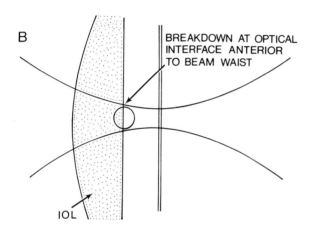

10. *Uncorrected chromatic aberration causes the Nd-YAG laser to focus at a location posterior to the He-Ne beam.* A simple lens brings shorter wavelengths to focus before longer wavelengths. Thus the He-Ne beam at 633 nm comes to a focal point that is anterior to the Nd-YAG radiation at 1064 nm. This concept ignores for the moment the variability of the location of optical breakdown due to other causes discussed earlier. A truly achromatic lens design, one without such chromatic aberration, is impossible to achieve over the entire spectrum but can be achieved for two specified wavelengths that are intended to be parfocal. The ophthalmic Nd-YAG laser should be designed and adjusted so that 633-nm and 1064-nm wavelengths are parfocal.

11. *The He-Ne focal point must be well defined.* The smaller the depth of focus of the He-Ne aiming beam, the more reproducible is the localization of the zone of the YAG optical breakdown. Objective measurements have shown that a well-defined dual He-Ne pattern has a smaller depth of focus than a number of alternative patterns, including a single beam or a ring.

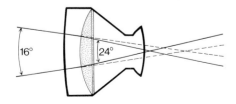

FIGURE 6–4

A contact lens with greater plus power than the corneal curvature results in increased convergence of the beam, a smaller focal spot size, and a magnified view for the surgeon, all of which improve critical focus. An increase in convergence angle from 16 to 24 degrees is illustrated.

TABLE 6–1. PRINCIPLES OF CRITICAL FOCUS

1. Optical breakdown is a nonlinear process.
2. Increasing energy input causes the breakdown zone to move anteriorly.
3. Using the minimum necessary energy helps to keep the He-Ne and YAG lasers parfocal.
4. The smaller the beam cone angle, the greater will be the anterior movement of a suprathreshold breakdown zone.
5. Suprathreshold energies result in an elongated breakdown region that extends anteriorly along the laser beam axis.
6. Predictable optical breakdown is degraded by media opacity.
7. Predictable optical breakdown is degraded by induced astigmatism.
8. The threshold for optical breakdown is lower at optical interfaces than in optically uniform media.
9. Use of a contact lens may enhance critical focus.
10. Uncorrected chromatic aberration causes the Nd-YAG laser to focus at a location posterior to the He-Ne beam.
11. The He-Ne focal point must be well defined.

TABLE 6–2. LASER DESIGN ELEMENTS THAT ENHANCE CRITICAL FOCUS

1. Large cone angle of converging laser light
2. Minimal focal spot size
3. Achromatic lens design
4. Infinitely adjustable energy selection
5. Coaxial slit lamp biomicroscope and laser beam optical pathway
6. Well-defined He-Ne focal point

Before using the laser each day the surgeon must perform a test of the delivery system optics. The oculars of the biomicroscope are adjusted, moving from plus ($+$) to minus ($-$), so that the biomicroscope, the slit illumination beam, and the He-Ne beam are all parfocal. By aiming the laser at a test object, at the minimum energy for reliable breakdown, the position of maximum optical breakdown is evaluated. If this position is not parfocal with the He-Ne beam, note of the position should be made until a laser adjustment can be achieved. The laser should not be used if grossly inaccurate YAG breakdown occurs. While the ideal test object is a thin membrane in a saline solution chamber, a tissue box wedged between the chin rest and forehead strap is a readily available substitute.

No artificial system can duplicate all of the variables in a given ophthalmic clinical application. Therefore, the initial shots in the patient's eyes should be made with particular caution and in a noncritical location. For example, the first shot of a posterior capsulotomy in the presence of a posterior chamber IOL should be in the periphery and never in the center of the optical axis (see the techniques discussed in Chapter 7).

The principles of critical focus are listed in Table 6–1. Table 6–2 summarizes the elements of laser design that enhance critical focus, and Table 6–3 lists the key elements for optimizing critical focus in typical clinical applications.

TABLE 6–3. ELEMENTS FOR OPTIMIZING SURGICAL CRITICAL FOCUS

1. The slit lamp and laser parfocality must be adjusted before beginning treatment.
2. The minimal amount of energy necessary should be used.
3. A contact lens should be employed as needed to improve stability, visualization, and optical breakdown localization.
4. The laser beam should be directed perpendicularly through the IOL and the central clear cornea.
5. The presence of nearby optical interfaces should be noted, especially posterior chamber implants during capsulotomy and the corneal endothelium in peripheral anterior chamber treatments.

7

POSTERIOR CAPSULOTOMY AND PUPILLARY MEMBRANECTOMY

The Q-switched and mode-locked Nd-YAG lasers have rapidly entered the ophthalmic surgical armamentarium as the tools of choice for discission of the posterior capsule.[1-3] For a new and costly technology, the purchase and application of these lasers have occurred at an unprecedented rate. The large shift in the past decade from intracapsular to extracapsular surgery generated a widespread need for safe and effective techniques to manage both intact posterior capsules that opacify postoperatively and visually significant capsular fragments that remain after primary surgical capsular discission.

EXTRACAPSULAR SURGERY AND THE POSTERIOR CAPSULE

RATIONALE

A brief review of the rationale for extracapsular surgery and secondary laser capsulotomy is appropriate.

Cystoid Macular Edema. The rate of persistent postoperative cystoid macular edema (CME) has been the focus of several studies comparing intracapsular and extracapsular cataract extraction. Jaffe, Clayman, and co-workers have reported an ongoing study of a series of patients with cataract surgery and intraocular lenses (IOLs) who had fluorescein angiographic follow-up one or more years after surgery.[4] In cases with an iris-fixated IOL, the prevalence of CME determined 16 to 24 months postoperatively was 15.4 per cent for intracapsular cataract extractions (ICCE) compared with 4.5 per cent for extracapsular cataract extractions (ECCE) involving intact capsules. A control group of IOL-eligible patients who declined an implant and underwent ICCE had a CME incidence rate of 8.5 per cent.

A subsequent series of operations was performed by the same surgeons using ECCE, Shearing posterior chamber IOL implant (PC IOL), and primary capsulotomy.[5] The long-term CME incidence rate was 3.0 per cent. Statistical analysis revealed differences in CME prevalence detected by fluorescein angiography at a level of $p < 0.05$ for each ECCE series compared with each ICCE series.

When the researchers analyzed "clinical" CME (which was undefined), the prevalence for the uncomplicated ECCE groups was zero. However, the

ICCE–iris-fixated IOL group had a prevalence of long-term clinical CME of 3.4 per cent, which was significantly higher than in the combined ECCE groups. The ICCE group without IOL had a prevalence of long-term "clinical" CME of 2.1 per cent. It was calculated that the vitreous loss rate in ECCE would have to be 20 per cent before fluorescein and clinical CME rates equalled the rates for ICCE with a vitreous loss rate of 3 per cent.[6] Similarly, Wetzig and coworkers found a CME rate of 8 per cent for ICCE compared with 1.2 per cent for ECCE.[7] When comparing any two series of patients, only one variable should differ; in particular, IOL type as well as surgical technique may heavily influence CME incidence.

With ECCE, CME may be reduced by leaving the capsule intact at the time of surgery, according to some studies. A review by Chambless of 1055 phacoemulsification ECCE patients found a reduced rate of clinical CME when the capsule remained intact (0.9 per cent) compared with open capsules (7.3 per cent).[8] Most open capsules were either cases early in the series or complicated cases. Primary and secondary discissions resulted in similar CME rates. In contrast, in a series of 450 ECCE cases, Emery found long-term clinical CME in 1 per cent of patients with intact capsules, in 1.4 per cent with secondary capsulotomy, and in 7 per cent with primary capsulotomy.[9]

A major prospective masked study of 288 patients by Kraff, Sanders, Jampol, and Lieberman further supports the concept of the beneficial role of an intact posterior capsule.[10] In uncomplicated ECCE cases, after the point of PC IOL insertion, patients were randomly assigned to either a group with intact capsules or one with primary bent needle central capsulotomy. At three to six months postoperatively masked fluorescein angiography was performed on all available patients (63 per cent). A statistically significant difference was found in the incidence of angiographically demonstrated CME of 21.5 per cent for the primary discission group compared with 5.6 per cent for the intact capsule group ($p = 0.003$). When CME occurred, it was milder in the intact capsule group compared with the primary capsulotomy group. In the primary capsulotomy group CME was associated with significantly poorer visual acuity ($p = 0.04$), whereas in the intact capsule group the occurrence of CME did not result in a significant reduction in visual acuity ($p = 0.25$).

In Lyle's series, the incidence of clinical CME was 8.3 per cent for ICCE, 0.8 per cent for ECCE with an intact capsule, and 1.7 per cent for ECCE with an open capsule.[11] However, statistical analysis was not provided, the type of capsulotomy was unspecified, and the follow-up period varied widely. In contrast, Sorr, Everett, and Hurite found the same 22 per cent incidence of fluorescein-positive subclinical CME within six weeks after ECCE whether the posterior capsule was intact or primary capsulotomy was performed.[12] Long-term follow-up was incomplete, however.

Retinal Detachment. The incidence of retinal detachment after cataract extraction is generally estimated to be between 1 and 3 per cent, with somewhat lower rates in some modern extracapsular series compared historically or retrospectively with intracapsular series.[11, 13–16] Jaffe, Clayman, and Jaffe compared the incidence of retinal detachment in two consecutive series of moderate to severe myopes who underwent ICCE or ECCE with an intact posterior capsule.[17] Follow-up ranged from one to four years, with an average of 2.8 years for both groups. In cases without vitreous loss, retinal detachment occurred in 7 of 122 ICCE patients (5.7 per cent) and one of 151 ECCE patients (0.7 per cent). The difference in this incidence was statistically significant ($p = 0.032$). In a series of 819 patients who underwent ICCE with iris plane IOLs, with a minimum two-year follow-up period, the incidence of retinal detachment rose from 0.7 per cent when globe axial length was less than 25 mm to 5 per cent when axial length was greater than 25 mm (difference significant at $= 0.05$).[14]

FIGURE 7–1

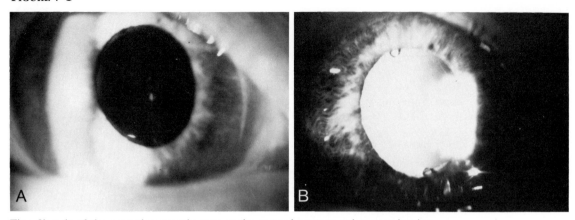

Fine fibrosis of the posterior capsule seen at the second postoperative examination represents cortical lamellae left at the time of surgery. The fibrosis is evident with oblique slit lamp illumination *(A)* but is optically insignificant when viewed with a red reflex *(B)*.

CAPSULAR OPACIFICATION

Postoperative opacification of initially clear posterior capsules occurs frequently in patients after extracapsular extraction of senile cataracts. Sinskey reported that 43 per cent of his patients required discission with an average follow-up of 26 months.[18] Emery found opacification in 28 per cent of patients with two to three years' follow-up.[19]

In adults, the time from surgery to visually significant opacification varies from months to years.[20] In younger age groups, almost 100 per cent opacification occurs within two years after surgery; in adults, the rate declines with increasing age.[19]

Clinically, optical degradation of initially clear posterior capsules takes several forms. *Fibrosis* connotes a gray white band or plaquelike opacity that usually is recognized in the early postoperative period. Fibrosis present in the first days to weeks postoperatively probably most often represents cortical lamellae left at the time of surgery (Fig. 7–1A, B). Fibrosis that develops months to years postoperatively is caused by multiple layers of anterior lens epithelium that have migrated and undergone fibrous metaplasia.[21] Figure 7–2 shows a dense fibrous plaque. Heavy fibrosis occurs frequently at the edge of a PC IOL placed in the bag with apposition of anterior and posterior capsules (Fig. 7–3).

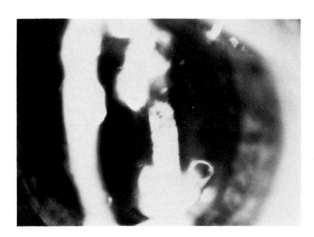

FIGURE 7–2

Heavy diffuse fibrosis of a posterior capsule behind a PC IOL.

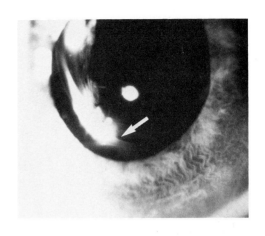

FIGURE 7–3

Dense fibrosis at the edge of a PC IOL optic placed in the bag *(arrow)*, in which an anterior capsular flap is apposed to the posterior capsule.

Migration of epithelial cells with formation of small *Elschnig's pearls* and *bladder cells,* the second major form of opacity, occurs months to years after surgery (Fig. 7–4). Pathologic examination indicates that the proliferating anterior epithelial cells originate at the site of apposition of the anterior capsular flaps to the posterior capsule.[21] This finding explains the inability of polishing of the capsule at surgery to delay the onset or reduce the frequency of late capsular opacification,[18, 20] because polishing of the posterior capsule cannot remove the epithelial cells from the anterior capsular flaps. Wide anterior capsulotomy may help to delay posterior capsular opacification by increasing the distance from the visual axis to the anterior capsular flaps. Mitotic inhibitors instilled into the anterior chamber after ECCE have been shown experimentally to dramatically reduce capsular opacification.[22]

Capsular wrinkling can have two manifestations. Broad undulations of clear capsule are particularly common in the early postoperative period before the capsule becomes tense. Posterior chamber lens haptics may induce these broad wrinkles along the axis of the haptic orientation. Conversely, a posterior chamber lens may tend to flatten broad wrinkles if the optic body or a YAG spacer bar or tab presses on the capsule (see Chapter 8). Fibrotic contraction can also induce broad wrinkles (Fig. 7–5). Broad undulating wrinkles of clear capsule rarely are visually disturbing to the patient; an unusual patient may perceive linear distortions or shadows that correspond to the wrinkles and are relieved by capsulotomy.

Fine wrinkles or folds in the capsule, in contrast, can result in marked optical disturbance (Fig. 7–6). These fine wrinkles are caused by myofibroblastic

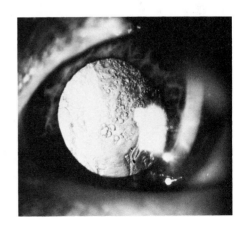

FIGURE 7–4

Red reflex view shows formation of multiple small epithelial pearls after anterior epithelial cells migrate centrally from peripheral areas of apposition of anterior capsular flaps to the posterior capsule.

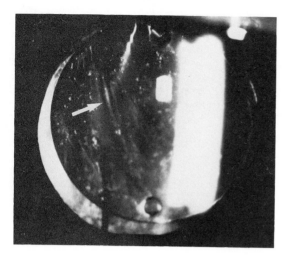

FIGURE 7–5

Broad wrinkles of the clear posterior capsule *(arrow)* are seen on red reflex, with numerous small epithelial pearls.

differentiation of the migrating lens epithelial cells, which acquire contractile properties, resulting in the wrinkles.[21]

If the iris forms synechiae to the capsule, reactive pigment epithelial hyperplasia and migration onto the capsule may occur. Most often these adhesions occur if large amounts of cortex are left at the time of surgery, which is particularly common with traumatic cataracts. Figure 7–7 shows dense melanin deposition on a pupillary membrane after an old traumatic cataract. Localized pigmented precipitates on the capsule and IOL can occur spontaneously or after hemorrhage or inflammation.

COMPLICATIONS OF SURGICAL POSTERIOR CAPSULAR DISCISSION

The data regarding a reduced incidence of CME with an intact posterior capsule compared with ECCE and primary capsulotomy already have been reviewed. With a rate of subsequent secondary capsulotomy as high as 50 per cent, however, and the high cost of Nd-YAG ophthalmic lasers, alternative methods and complications of secondary capsulotomy must be carefully considered.

Surgical secondary capsulotomy may be performed in several ways. In the office, the most common approach is with a fine needle or needle knife that is

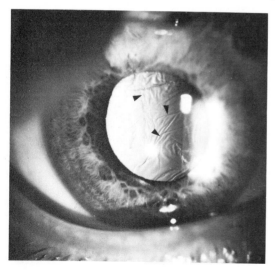

FIGURE 7–6

Fine wrinkles in the posterior capsule are evident on red reflex *(arrowheads)*. These wrinkles alone can be visually disturbing and reduce acuity by several lines.

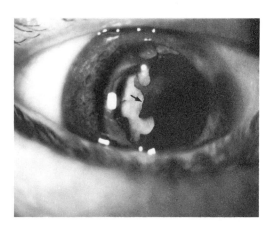

FIGURE 7–7

Pigment from proliferating uveal melanocytes has covered a large portion of this dense pupillary membrane, which formed after a traumatic cataract 40 years previously. The border of the pigment has a sharp scalloped configuration *(arrow)*.

passed through the limbus at the slit lamp or under an operating microscope with topical anesthesia.[23] In the operating room, alternative procedures include use of a knife or a vitrectomy instrument introduced through the limbus or pars plana.[24] The difficulty of passing an instrument behind a PC IOL to obtain a well-centered capsulotomy by the limbal approach has led some surgeons to advocate the routine use of the pars plana approach.[25] However, of these techniques, only that employing a bent needle that is passed through the limbus offers the potential for not violating the anterior hyaloid face.

Lindstrom and Harris reported 42 posterior capsule discissions performed through the pars plana in the presence of a PC IOL.[25] Cystoid macular edema associated with visual acuity of less than 20/40 was recognized in four patients after discission (9.5 per cent); three cases resolved (criterion for resolution, time course, and final acuity were undefined), and one case persisted with visual acuity between 20/80 and 20/200. One retinal detachment caused by a single horseshoe tear was diagnosed five months after capsulotomy and 17 months after cataract surgery. One IOL subluxated and required operative repositioning. All cases of CME occurred in patients with capsulotomy performed within one year after cataract surgery, and in three of the four cases less than six months had elapsed between cataract extraction and discission. Only half of the discissions were performed on patients within the first postoperative year, and the absence of complications in patients with more than one year between ECCE and discission led to a widely cited recommendation that surgical discission be deferred for at least a year after ECCE. Statistical analysis of results was not given.

While it is plausible that a more recently operated eye is more vulnerable to CME induced by a surgical discission, it is possible that the CME was present before capsulotomy and that the visual impairment was mistakenly attributed to the presence of the capsule. Alternatively, patients with early capsular opacification may not represent a population equivalent to those with late opacification. A number of interacting variables may be present, including age, surgical trauma, and the presence of lens remnants and their inflammatory potential. Jaffe believes that the patients with late capsular opacification are those with a smooth postoperative course and little inflammation.[26]

Livernois and Sinskey reported 142 secondary capsulotomies made by a limbal approach.[27] All operations were done later than six months after ECCE. In one of 41 aphakic eyes and four of 101 pseudophakic eyes clinically recognized CME developed and was confirmed by fluorescein angiography, for an overall incidence of 3.5 per cent. The condition of only one patient, who had pseudophakia, eventually improved during the minimum follow-up period of 18 months. Two other cases developed a severe postcapsulotomy inflammatory response.

McPherson, O'Malley, and Bravo studied 27 cases of retinal detachment in eyes with ECCE and secondary surgical discission.[28] In the cases of only four eyes did less than one year elapse between cataract extraction and discission. Visual outcome was poorer for this group, with only one of four attaining vision of 20/400 or better, compared with 22 of 23 eyes with more than one year between cataract surgery and discission. Detachments occurring within one year after discission were more extensive, but visual outcome was better than for detachments occurring more than one year after discission. Typical breaks involved one or two small horseshoe tears somewhat more likely to occur inferiorly than superiorly. No data on the fellow eye were given, and no statistical analysis of these comparisons was reported.

RESULTS AND COMPLICATIONS FROM Nd-YAG LASER POSTERIOR CAPSULOTOMY

The initial European response to experience with Q-switched and mode-locked Nd-YAG laser secondary capsulotomy in large numbers of patients has been enthusiastic.[1-3] Early short-term American experience has also demonstrated the relative ease of laser capsulotomy with a high rate of visual improvement, but not without complications, including acute transient pressure rise, IOL marking, rupture of the anterior hyaloid face, retinal detachment, and bleeding from diabetic rubeosis iridis.[29-31]

Keates, Steinert, Puliafito, and Maxwell reported the results of a study of 526 patients who underwent Q-switched Nd-YAG laser posterior capsulotomy and were followed a minimum of six months by their physicians.[32] These results were compared with observations of a historical control group of 209 pseudophakes who had undergone surgical secondary capsulotomy before the laser became available. The surgical control population had significantly better prediscission visual acuity and lesser preoperative pathology. Nevertheless, 85.7 per cent of the laser-treated pseudophakes achieved 20/40 or better vision compared with 80.2 per cent of the surgically treated group. Excluding patients with preoperative pathology, 90.1 per cent of the laser-treated pseudophakes obtained better vision after treatment, compared with 69.7 per cent of the surgically treated pseudophakes (difference significant at $p<0.001$).

Of the laser-treated pseudophakes, 3.3 per cent had diminished vision after capsulotomy, compared with 14.8 per cent of the surgical control group ($p<0.001$). Half of the patients in the laser-treated group with diminished posttreatment acuity at six months were within one line of their pretreatment visual acuity. Cystoid macular edema was diagnosed at any one of the posttreatment visits in 2.3 per cent of the patients, but at six months persistent CME was reported in only one patient (0.2 per cent). This was significantly less than the persistent CME rate for the surgical control group of 1.9 per cent ($p<0.05$). Retinal detachment occurred in two of the laser-treated (0.4 per cent) and in none of the surgically treated patients. Persistent pressure elevation, iritis, vitritis, anterior segment hemorrhage, and IOL dislocation were all reported in fewer than 1 per cent of patients. IOL marks were reported for 33 per cent of patients with posterior chamber lenses, 4.3 per cent with iris lenses, and 6.5 per cent with anterior chamber lenses.

Pressure Elevation After Laser Capsulotomy. Posttreatment pressure elevation is now recognized as a common, although usually transient, complication after Nd-YAG laser capsulotomy. In a report of 49 capsulotomies, Terry, Stark, Maumenee, and Fagadau detected a pressure increase in 37 eyes, with a maximal pressure greater than 30 mm Hg in 16 eyes and greater than 50 mm Hg in four eyes.[29] In most eyes the pressure returned to pretreatment levels within one week, but in two eyes it did not normalize until six weeks after treatment. When patients were observed carefully after laser capsulotomy, the majority were found to have a pressure peak within three hours after the operation. Channell and Beckman found a pressure elevation exceeding 5 mm Hg in 64 per cent of patients and 10 mm Hg in 35 per cent of patients within four hours of laser capsulotomy.[33] Persistent pressure elevation after one month occurred in 5 per cent.

Richter, Arzeno, Pappas, and coworkers examined the acute elevation of pressure after laser capsulotomy with serial pressure measurements and tonography in 17 patients.[34] The median time to achieve maximal pressure was three hours. The higher the pretreatment intraocular pressure and the lower the pretreatment facility of outflow, the greater was the tendency for a large pressure increase. As a consequence, patients with pre-existing open angle glaucoma had a higher risk of developing greater pressure elevation. A decline in the facility of outflow paralleled any acute rise in pressure after laser capsulotomy, and the outflow facility returned to baseline level as the pressure normalized.

Mechanistically, the acute pressure rise is thus caused by impaired outflow, and the rapid onset suggests that the reduced outflow may be related to capsular debris, acute inflammatory cells, heavy molecular-weight protein, or a combination of these mechanisms.[35] An immunologic reaction to liberated lens proteins is unlikely to have such a rapid onset and resolution.

In this small series,[34] patients with IOLs in any location tended to have a smaller elevation in pressure. Such a finding has been noted anecdotally by many clinicians, particularly with posterior chamber lenses. This effect may be related to posterior trapping of capsular debris by the IOL. Alternatively, patients with IOLs may have capsule characteristics different from aphakes, either because of the IOL itself or because of different visual expectations for IOL patients, which lead to capsulotomy at an earlier stage, with less fibrotic material or pearl formation. Other investigators have not found a significant difference in the extent of pressure elevation in the presence of IOLs.[33]

Variables that did not predict a postcapsulotomy pressure rise included use of systemic anti-inflammatory agents for other disorders (such as arthritis), the degree of capsular opacity, the laser pulse energy, the number of shots, the total energy delivered, and the amount of anterior chamber cell and debris as judged at the slit lamp.

In this study,[34] measurement of the pressure at one hour could accurately predict the ultimate rise in pressure. If at one hour the pressure increase had already exceeded the baseline measurement by more than 5 mm Hg, there was an eventual total increase in excess of 10 mm Hg. A one-hour pressure increase less than 5 mm Hg reliably predicted a maximum pressure increase of under 10 mm Hg. Occasionally, however, pressure elevation may be delayed in onset and missed if checked only at one hour.[33]

These findings are in agreement with the statistical analysis of the core study data by Keates and coworkers.[32] In that study, preoperative glaucoma or preoperative pressure of greater than 20 mm Hg predicted a higher chance of postoperative pressure increase above 30 mm Hg. Glaucoma patients with preoperative pressure greater than 20 mm Hg were eight times more likely to have increases above 30 mm Hg than were nonglaucomatous patients with baseline pressure below 20 mm Hg. The incidence of persistent elevation of pressure six months after treatment was 0.8 per cent.

TECHNIQUE FOR POSTERIOR CAPSULOTOMY

Preoperative Assessment. All patients require a complete ophthalmic history and examination before treatment, including notation of medical history, topical and systemic medications, vision, intraocular pressure in both eyes, slit lamp examination, and fundus examination. Judging the contribution of a

TABLE 7–1. ASSESSMENT OF OPTICAL SIGNIFICANCE OF CAPSULAR OPACITY

1. Direct ophthalmoscopic visualization of fundus structures
2. Retinoscopy
3. Red reflex evaluation by
   a. Slit lamp examination
   b. Direct ophthalmoscopic examination
   c. Indirect ophthalmoscopic examination
4. Hruby lens view of fundus
5. Laser interferometer evaluation
6. Potential Acuity Meter evaluation
7. Fluorescein angiography or angioscopy

capsular opacity to the patient's overall visual deficit may be difficult. Table 7–1 lists useful techniques. Some capsular opacities are impressive in oblique slit lamp illumination but are insignificant when viewed against the red reflex. In general, these opacities cause little visual difficulty. The single most reliable technique for assessing capsular opacity is direct ophthalmoscopy, since visibility of retinal details correlates with the patient's view of the world. Retinoscopy and the red reflex seen at the slit lamp or with a direct or indirect ophthalmoscope also reveal significant optical disturbances. The fundus view with the Hruby lens may also allow accurate assessment of capsular clouding, whereas the indirect ophthalmoscope can penetrate significant capsular opacity.

The laser interferometer and the Potential Acuity Meter should penetrate mild to moderate capsular opacity and indicate macular function. Both instruments may give false-positive ("good") acuity prediction in the presence of cystoid macular edema,[36]* which is the most likely cause of postcataract visual impairment besides capsular opacity itself.

Unless the capsule is extremely dense, adequate visualization may be present for fluorescein angiography or angioscopy. In patients in whom the capsular opacity seems inadequate to explain the quality of vision, CME should be anticipated and documented, so that unnecessary and possibly deleterious capsulotomy can be avoided.

Preparation of the Patient. *Dilation* of the pupil facilitates visualization of the capsule over a broad expanse. Except in the case of an iris-clip lens, dilation is very helpful for a surgeon inexperienced with laser capsulotomy. In the absence of a miotic pupil, however, dilation may be omitted. The possible role of cycloplegia in the post–laser-treatment pressure increase has not yet been studied.

If the pupil is to be dilated, the landmarks of the pupillary zone of the capsule should be sketched beforehand. Pupils are often eccentric or may dilate eccentrically, as shown in Figure 7–8. Inattention to the pupillary zone results in an eccentric capsulotomy and may necessitate a second session at the laser or induce the surgeon to perform an overly large capsulotomy to prevent this possibility. If the laser is available, the patient can be brought to the laser before dilation, and a single *"marker" shot* can be placed in the capsule near the middle of the pupillary axis. When the pupil is subsequently dilated, the marker shot accurately reminds the surgeon of the patient's true visual axis.

For routine dilation, the authors recommend only a single drop of 2.5 per cent phenylephrine. If this is inadequate, a drop of 0.5 or 1 per cent tropicamide may be added. Weak dilation is intended to prevent inadvertent iris capture of a PC IOL (Fig. 7–9), which may be difficult to properly reposition.

Figure 7–10 shows an example of a posterior capsulotomy performed without dilation. As the patient looks up, down, left, and right, the laser can be applied to capsular edges behind the sphincter, so the capsulotomy can be

---

*JM Minkowski 1983: personal communication.

FIGURE 7–8

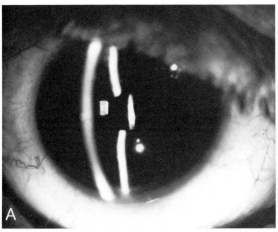 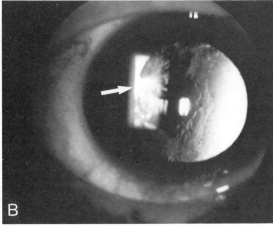

(A) Typical capsular opacity before dilation. *(B)* Capsulotomy appears eccentric because of uneven pupillary dilation caused by posterior synechia to the capsule *(arrow)*. The capsular opening is properly centered for the undilated pupil.

perfectly centered. The slit lamp illumination should be with a narrow beam, angled obliquely, to minimize miosis and indicate average pupillary size with ambient lighting.

The purpose and nature of the procedure should be explained to the patient and informed consent obtained beforehand, if at all possible. At the time of treatment, the patient usually is reassured by the familiar appearance of the slit lamp delivery system. The surgeon should remind the patient that the procedure is painless. The patient may hear small clicks or pops, but the patient must simply maintain steady fixation. The procedure is completed in a matter of minutes.

No anesthesia is generally required for capsulotomy unless a contact lens is employed. In that case, a drop of topical anesthetic is applied to the cornea immediately before the beginning of the procedure. In rare circumstances, such as nystagmus, a retrobulbar injection for akinesia may be helpful. If topical anesthetic is applied in advance of the procedure for examination or instillation of painful mydriatics and cycloplegics, the patient should be instructed to keep

FIGURE 7–9

Iris capture of a ciliary sulcus fixated planar haptic PC IOL. This phenomenon can occur after wide dilation for posterior capsulotomy. If dilation is necessary at all, weak mydriatics and cycloplegics should be employed.

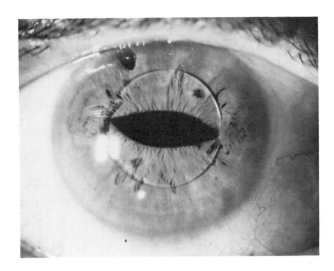

FIGURE 7–10

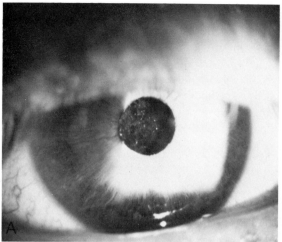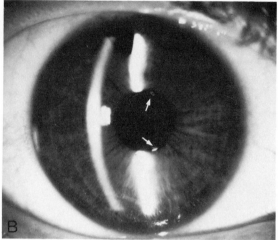

Posterior capsulotomy performed without pupillary dilation. *(A)* Hazy capsule before treatment. *(B)* After laster application the pupillary zone is clear. Two tags of capsule at the edge of the pupil can be seen *(arrows)*. These could be easily exposed to the laser by having the patient look up and down.

the eyes closed during the interval while waiting for the laser treatment, in order to maintain the surface integrity and optical quality of the corneal epithelium.

The patient must be seated comfortably with properly adjusted stool, table, and chin rest heights and a foot rest when appropriate. A strap that passes from the headrest behind the patient's head is useful to counteract the tendency of many patients to move back during the course of the treatment. The surgeon's visualization of the target is usually improved in a darkened room. If the patient is expected to fixate with the other eye, however, an illuminated fixation target should be provided.

Table 7–2 summarizes the steps in patient preparation.

Contraindications. Attempted Nd-YAG laser capsulotomy is contraindicated if corneal scars, irregularity, or edema preclude adequate visualization of the target or degrade the laser beam optics to prevent reliable and predictable optical breakdown. The procedure is also contraindicated if the patient proves unable or unwilling to fixate adequately, with the threat of inadvertent damage to adjacent intraocular structures.

TABLE 7–2. PREPARATION OF THE PATIENT

Before the treatment session
1. Complete ophthalmic history and examination.
2. Discussion of proposed procedure, including risks, benefits, and alternatives; signing of informed consent form
3. Pupillary dilation (optional)
   a. Determination of visual axis and normal pupillary size: sketch and preliminary laser marker shot
   b. Weak mydriatics and cycloplegics: 2.5% phenylephrine or 0.5% or 1% tropicamide

At the laser
1. Review of the procedure, the expected pop or click, and the importance of fixation
2. Application of topical anesthetic if contact lens is to be used
3. Adjustment of stool, table, chin rest, and foot rest for optimal patient comfort
4. Application of head strap to maintain forehead position
5. Darkening of the room (optional)
6. Provision of fixation target for fellow eye (illumination of target if room is darkened)

TABLE 7–3. CONTRAINDICATIONS TO LASER CAPSULOTOMY

Absolute contraindications
1. Corneal scars, irregularities, or edema that:
    a. Interfere with target visualization
    b. Make optical breakdown unpredictable
2. Inadequate stability of the eye

Relative contraindications
1. Glass IOL
2. Known or suspected CME
3. Active intraocular inflammation
4. High risk for retinal detachment

The presence of a glass intraocular lens is a relative contraindication. The merits of surgical discission in this instance should be carefully weighed. Laser capsulotomy should be approached with extreme caution and only by an experienced YAG laser operator under ideal conditions, because of the possibility of causing a complete fracture in the glass optic.[37]

Known or suspected cystoid macular edema is a relative contraindication, given current evidence regarding a possible beneficial effect from an intact posterior capsule and in view of rare cases of clinical CME that apparently occur after Nd-YAG laser capsulotomy.[32]

Unlike the situation with surgical discission, the only data available to date do not show a difference in the rate of complications depending on the interval between cataract surgery and laser capsulotomy.[32] However, given the overall low incidence of long-term complications, recognition of such a trend may require an even larger study. Conservative practice suggests avoidance of capsulotomy in an eye with active inflammation until the visual impairment becomes functionally unacceptable to the patient.

No data exist on laser capsulotomy in eyes at high risk for retinal detachment. As a minimal precaution, the least amount of energy and the lowest number of shots should be used that can accomplish the capsulotomy, and only a small opening should be made. The alternative of repolishing the capsule should be considered.

Table 7–3 summarizes the absolute and relative contraindications to laser capsulotomy.

Capsulotomy Technique. The minimal amount of energy necessary to obtain breakdown and rupture the capsule is desired. With most lasers, a typical capsule can be opened by using 1 to 2 mJ per pulse.

The capsule is examined for wrinkles that indicate tension lines. Shots placed across tension lines result in the largest opening per pulse, since the tension causes the initial opening to widen.

Figure 7–11 shows an actual capsulotomy photographed sequentially and drawn from the photographs, showing the opening as it develops and the location of the next laser shot. Table 7–4 outlines the basic technique. The usual strategy is to create a cruciate opening, beginning superiorly near the 12

TABLE 7–4. POSTERIOR CAPSULOTOMY TECHNIQUE

1. Use minimum energy:
    1 mJ if possible.
2. Identify and cut across tension lines.
3. Perform a cruciate opening:
    Begin in 12 o'clock periphery.
    Progress toward 6 o'clock position.
    Cut across at 3 and 9 o'clock positions.
    Clean up any residual tags.
    Avoid freely floating fragments.

FIGURE 7–11

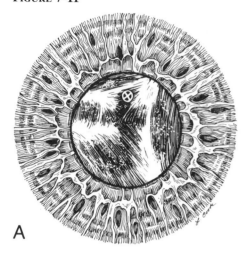

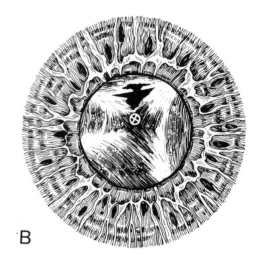

A

B

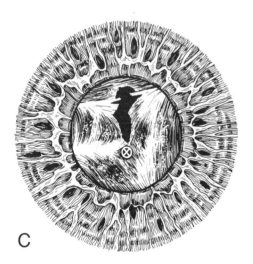

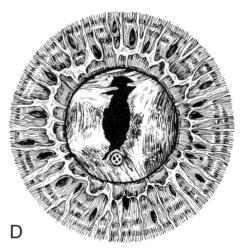

C

D

Artist's drawing based on sequential capsulotomy photographs. The capsulotomy is developed in a cruciate pattern. *(A)* The first shot is made superiorly in the location of some fine tension lines. *(B)* The second shot is aimed inside the inferior edge of the initial opening. *(C)* The next shot again is made at the 6 o'clock position of the capsulotomy border. *(D)* The fourth shot is made across inferior tension lines to allow the capsulotomy to widen.

FIGURE 7–11 *(Continued)*

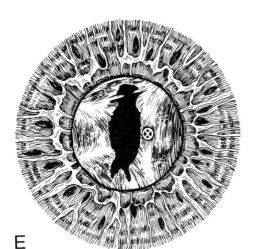

E

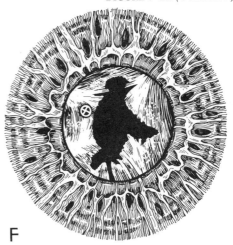

F

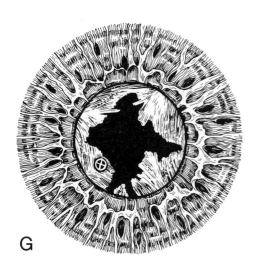

G

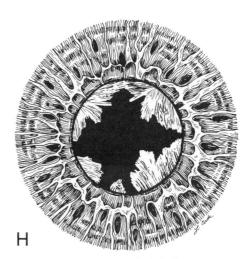

H

(E) The opening is nearly 3 mm wide. It is widened by a shot at the 3 o'clock capsulotomy margin. *(F)* The opening now needs to be directed to the left, with a shot at the 9 o'clock position. *(G)* The cruciate opening has been accomplished, but a triangular flap extends into the pupillary space from the 7:30 o'clock region in the left inferior pupil. A shot is applied to the flap, to both cut it and push it toward the periphery. *(H)* The capsulotomy is complete, and the pupil will be clear of capsule when the dilation wears off.

o'clock position and progressing downward toward the 6 o'clock position. Unless a wide opening has already developed, shots are then placed at the edge of the capsule opening, progressing laterally toward the 3 and 9 o'clock positions. If any capsular flaps remain in the pupillary space, the laser is fired specifically at the flaps to cut them and cause them to retract and fall back to the periphery.

The goal is to achieve flaps based in the periphery and inferiorly. Free-floating fragments should be avoided because these may remain and cause interference. Cutting in a circle, "can-opener style," should be avoided, since this tends to create large fragments that may not settle or that may settle against the endothelium or angle structures.

Beginning the cruciate opening in the superior periphery has several advantages. The initial shots are in the periphery so that if the patient startles and an adjacent IOL is marked, the mark appears in the periphery. Both patient and surgeon can have settled down before the more critical central area is treated. Furthermore, gravity aids in pulling the flaps, as they develop, toward the inferior periphery. In contrast, a flap hanging down from above can be much more difficult to cause to retract.

An IOL may be marked in the course of the capsulotomy. This is particularly true for posterior chamber lenses for which little or no separation of the capsule from the IOL exists. The issue of laser damage to the IOL and IOL designs for use with the YAG laser are discussed in detail in Chapter 8. Color Plate I*A* and Figure 7–12 show a capsulotomy without damage to an overlying PC IOL.

Visually significant pits and cracks can be minimized and avoided through careful techniques, as outlined in Table 7–5. The minimal amount of energy must be employed. With a typical capsule and careful focusing, 1.0 mJ is usually adequate. A contact lens such as the Peyman or central Abraham lens (see pp. 60–61) stabilizes the eye, improves the laser beam optics, and facilitates accurate focusing. The capsule should be carefully examined for an area of separation from the IOL in which to begin the capsulotomy. Once the capsulotomy has begun, further areas of separation usually develop.

Following the usual strategy of beginning the capsulotomy in the 12 o'clock periphery gives an indication of the tendency for IOL marking in a noncritical area. If there is a tendency for unavoidable repeated marks, the usual cruciate pattern should be modified. Instead of progressing from the 12 o'clock to the 6 o'clock positions across the visual axis, the cut should be made nasally and

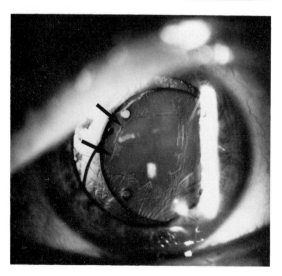

FIGURE 7–12

Posterior capsulotomy performed on a capsule in direct apposition to a lathe-cut PC IOL. Figure 7–6 is the pretreatment photograph of the same eye. Note the eccentric location of the optic caused by placement of the inferior haptic in the bag and the superior haptic in the ciliary sulcus. The capsulotomy is properly located in the visual axis, but care is taken to avoid opening beyond the edge of the optic so as to avoid vitreous herniation around the optic (*arrows*).

TABLE 7–5. Minimizing IOL Laser Marks

1. Use minimum energy.
2. Use a contact lens to:
     stabilize the eye.
     improve laser beam optics.
     facilitate accurate focusing.
3. Identify any areas of IOL-capsule separation, and begin treatment there.
4. If lens marking is occurring, make an opening in the shape of a Christmas tree from the 12 o'clock to the 4:30 o'clock positions and from the 12 o'clock to the 7:30 o'clock positions without placing any shots in the central optical zone.
5. Use deep-focus techniques:
     Optical breakdown occurs in the anterior vitreous.
     The shock wave radiates forward and ruptures the capsule.
     Higher energy (2 mJ or more) must be used.

temporally, staying in the periphery of the optical zone. The capsule then can be opened in a "Christmas-tree" fashion, based inferiorly, without any shots in the central visual axis.

One other technique is very helpful in avoiding IOL marks. The laser can be intentionally focused posteriorly to the capsule, to cause optical breakdown in the anterior vitreous. The shock wave then radiates forward and ruptures the capsule. Optical breakdown just at the capsule and IOL surface, with resultant IOL marking, is avoided. Because the breakdown threshold is higher in the uniform anterior vitreous than at an optical interface like the capsule, higher energy is required to use this technique, usually a minimum of 2 mJ. Therefore, care must be taken to consistently focus at an area posterior to the capsule, so that the breakdown is not allowed to come up to the back of the IOL, which would result in a larger mark (this phenomenon is discussed in Chapter 6). Because this technique traumatizes the vitreous, with as yet unknown long-term clinical significance, the authors prefer to avoid the deep-focus technique whenever possible.

In aphakes, the reverse of a deep-focus approach, namely deliberate focus anterior to the capsule, has been advocated by some as a mechanism for opening the capsule while leaving the anterior hyaloid intact. The clinical importance of an intact hyaloid after capsulotomy is unknown.

Capsulotomy Size. In the absence of a specific reason for a small opening, such as concern over a patient at high risk for retinal detachment, the capsulotomy should be as large as the pupil in ambient light. A small opening in a dense membrane results in excellent optics, analogous to those of a small pupil (see Fig. 7–15). When the capsule is only hazy and transmits images to the retina, however, a small opening is an improvement but is still suboptimal. The hazy membrane continues to transmit a poor-quality image that mixes with the image transmitted through the clear opening.

The percentage of the pupillary aperture that is cleared by capsulotomies of various sizes is given in Table 7–6, calculated for a 4-mm pupil. Maximal visual potential can be achieved only with full pupillary sized capsulotomy.

TABLE 7–6. Percentage of a 4-mm Pupillary Aperture That is Cleared by Capsulotomies of Different Sizes

Capsulotomy Diameter (mm)	Percentage Cleared (%)
1	6
2	25
3	56
4	100

A capsule with residual haze not only impairs vision under standard conditions but also produces glare. A clinical study of glare after ECCE substantiated the deleterious effect of capsular opacification.[38] The authors have studied this problem by constructing a camera in which the camera lens consists of an intraocular lens. Various pupillary conditions can then be modeled. Figure 7–13 shows a front-illuminated Snellen chart and an automobile headlight photographed through a hazy membrane with openings of various sizes. Glare and haze begin to diminish rapidly with 3 mm opening, but only with a full 4 mm opening do the glare and haze fully resolve.

FIGURE 7–13

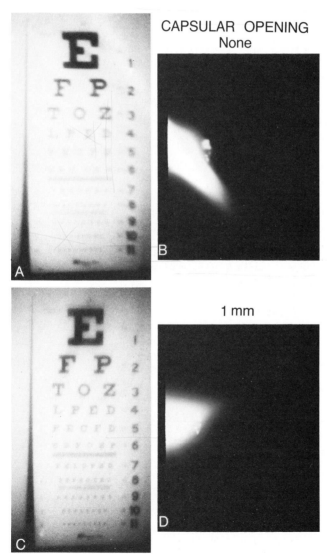

CAPSULAR OPENING
None

1 mm

FIGURE 7–13

Simulation of pseudophakic vision by a camera fitted with an IOL lens, a 4 mm "pupillary" aperture, and a hazy membrane "capsule." A front-illuminated Snellen chart is shown in the left column; a car headlight viewed obliquely is shown in the right column. The rows, as marked, progress from no opening, at the top, in 1 mm stages to a full 4 mm opening at the bottom. Only the full 4 mm opening is free of haze and glare, although smaller openings provide considerable improvement compared with the unopened capsule.

FIGURE 7–13 *(Continued)*

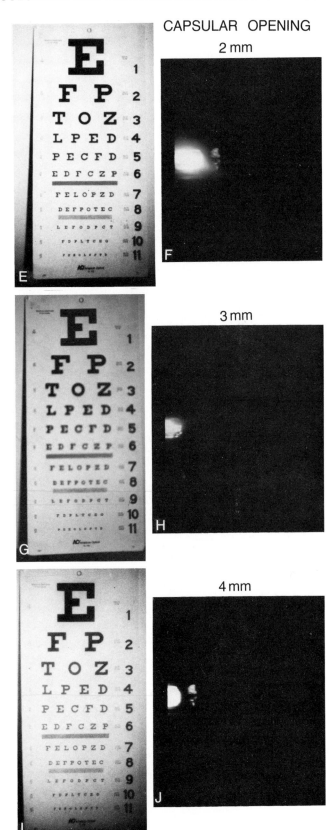

Postoperative Care. After laser capsulotomy, protocols for routine administration of topical steroids and cycloplegics vary widely according to the individual surgeon's clinical experience. The authors recommend routine use of topical steroids. The patient is discharged with instructions to apply a strong topical steroid (prednisolone 1 per cent or dexamethasone 0.1 per cent, for example) beginning immediately and continuing four times daily. This application is tapered and discontinued at postoperative visits when the clinical examination discloses an eye without cellular reaction.

As discussed earlier in this chapter, an acute increase in pressure in the hours after treatment is common. Ideally the patient is rechecked one hour and four hours after capsulotomy, and treatment is begun if the pressure has risen 5 or more mm Hg above baseline. If the patient cannot be checked until the next day, has a baseline pressure greater than 20 mm Hg, or has glaucoma, prophylactic treatment is given. Allergies and medical history must be reviewed. If there is no contraindication such as asthma or congestive heart disease, a drop of timolol 0.5 per cent at the conclusion of treatment usually suffices to blunt the pressure rise, since this medication has a maximal effect two to four hours after administration. Alternative medications are pilocarpine or a carbonic anhydrase inhibitor (of course, if the patient is cycloplegic administration of a miotic substance is less effective). The possibility of a delayed pressure elevation after use of these medications must be recognized. An examination on the day following laser treatment is indicated.

For patients already receiving medication for pre-existing glaucoma, the level of medication should be increased, using additional or stronger medication. If the patient is already on maximally tolerated medical therapy, a full dose (calculated by weight) of an oral osmotic agent (glycerin or isosorbide dinitrate) should be administered at the conclusion of the treatment and the patient instructed to take another full dose four hours after treatment.

Glaucoma patients on intensive therapy, particularly with advanced visual field loss, should be observed closely for at least four to six hours after treatment. Further options for management of sight-threatening pressure elevation include, progressively, intravenous administration of mannitol, anterior chamber paracentesis, anterior chamber washout, and emergency filtration. A case of postcapsulotomy intraocular pressure rise above 80 mm Hg with loss of light perception was successfully treated with anterior chamber paracentesis, and visual recovery to 20/25 was achieved.[39] Treatment of these high-risk patients may be less hazardous if the treatment is divided across multiple sessions, with a few shots given at low energy per session. However, studies of

TABLE 7–7. POSTCAPSULOTOMY CARE

Medication
A. Cycloplegics (optional)
   1% cyclopentolate at time of treatment
B. Steroids
   1% prednisolone or 0.1% dexamethasone four times a day, tapered as needed
C. Antiglaucoma medications
   Timolol 0.5% at time of treatment and as needed
   Pilocarpine 2 to 4% at time of treatment and as needed
   Carbonic anhydrase inhibitor at time of treatment and as needed
Minimal suggested follow-up protocol
A. One to four hours
   Pressure rise of 5 mm Hg: treatment should be given
B. One day
C. One week
D. One month
E. Three months
F. Six months

capsulotomy in the general population have not found a correlation of pressure increase with pulse energy, total shots, or total energy.[32, 34]

Two other causes of acute glaucoma after laser capsulotomy have been reported. Vitreous herniation may cause pupillary block and acute glaucoma.[40] In the absence of a patent peripheral iridectomy, the potential for pupillary block after posterior capsulotomy should be considered unless a posterior chamber lens is present that holds the vitreous in place. An aphakic iridectomy can be readily and safely performed with the YAG laser (see Chapter 9). A case of vitreous herniation plugging a filtering bleb with acute pressure increase ten days after capsulotomy has also been reported.[41]

The minimum follow-up requirements are based on the investigational protocol governing the use of the particular laser involved. Minimal suggested follow-up, whenever possible, is made at one to four hours, one day, one week, and one, three, and six months.

Table 7–7 summarizes typical postoperative care after laser capsulotomy.

TECHNIQUE FOR POSTERIOR MEMBRANECTOMY

Application of the Q-switched Nd-YAG laser to pupillary membranes was first described by Fankhauser et al.[42] While less common than posterior capsulotomy, the procedure offers the potential to optically clear the pupil in eyes that frequently have had serious pathology and are either poor candidates for further surgery or, if surgery were to be performed, require major procedures in the operating room with irrigation-suction-cutting instruments.

Several special aspects of the treatment of dense membranes must be considered.

Evaluation. The density and type of membrane should be evaluated to determine whether laser treatment is appropriate. Dense membranes may require multiple sessions to achieve an adequate opening, and the patient should be informed of this possibility. Lengthy sessions with many pulses and liberation of a large amount of debris seem prone to prolonged postlaser inflammation and elevated pressure. Large Elschnig's pearls, from old cataracts, when opened may liberate protein and result in phacoanaphylactic or phacolytic glaucoma. Such patients may be best served, in the end, by a definitive surgical operation instead of attempted laser membranectomy.

Membranectomy Technique. Unlike posterior capsules, in which each laser shot results in a large opening because the capsule is thin and under tension, membranes have little or no elastic properties. Treatment with the laser may require high pulse energy, from 4 to 12 mJ. The opening is created by "chipping" away at the edge, in a manner similar to that of a stonemason chipping at marble.

Figure 7–14 illustrates the case of an elderly woman who required cyclocryotherapy to control synechial angle closure glaucoma after penetrating keratoplasty for aphakic bullous keratoplasty. Subsequently an inflammatory membrane condensed across the pupil and reduced vision to hand motions. Her overall health as well as her ocular condition made her a poor risk for further surgery. When the Nd-YAG laser became available, the membrane was successfully opened. This required over 300 shots at up to 9 mJ. It is interesting that there was no pressure elevation—a finding that is consistent with the reduced aqueous production after cyclocryotherapy to compensate for already severely impaired outflow. There was no trabecular meshwork to be obstructed by protein and debris. Vision improved to 20/70, and the operated eye became the patient's better eye.

FIGURE 7–14

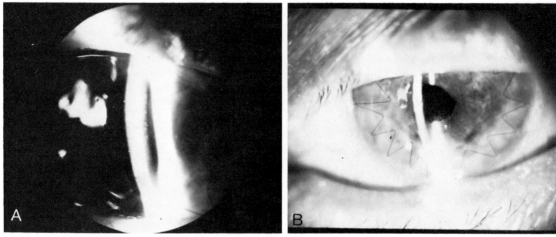

(A) Inflammatory pupillary membrane in a patient who required cyclocryotherapy for uncontrolled glaucoma after penetrating keratoplasty for aphakic bullous keratopathy. Visual acuity was limited to hand motions. (B) A 3 mm membranectomy by the Q-switched Nd-YAG laser, requiring over 300 shots at up to 9 mJ. Vision improved to 20/70.

FIGURE 7–15

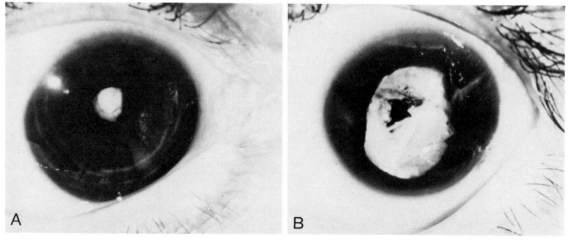

(A) Dense retropupillary membrane after complicated ECCE. (B) An adequate membrane opening is well centered on the pupillary axis.

FIGURE 7–16

An apparently eccentric opening is to compensate for an eccentric pupil caused by synechia to the area of penetrating injury at the limbus at 4 o'clock of the circumference. This case seen before treatment is shown in Figure 7–7. Note that the pressure waves have caused separation of the loosely adherent proliferating layer of melanocytes from the membrane *(arrow)*.

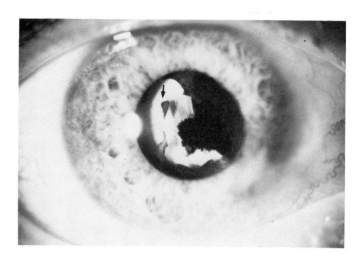

A small opening in a dense membrane can be quite satisfactory visually, as illustrated in Figure 7–15. Care must be taken to carefully center the opening within the pupil. The importance of careful positioning is also made by the case illustrated in Figure 7–16, in which the apparently eccentric opening is centered on the undilated pupil.

Retained cortical material may be treated with the laser before it condenses into a permanent membrane or to speed its eventual resorption. Figure 7–17 illustrates a case of ECCE with PC IOL in which an initially small amount of retained cortex at the 12 o'clock position swelled postoperatively to occlude the visual axis. When observed for several weeks, the material showed no evidence of resorption (Fig. 7–17A). The Nd-YAG laser set at 4 mJ was focused behind the IOL in the cortex and fired repeatedly in a procedure known as "corticolysis". The cortex became progressively "milky" with successive shots. After one week the pupillary zone had cleared (Fig. 7–17B). Prelaser visual acuity of hand motions improved to 20/30. The posterior capsule remained intact and clear.

FIGURE 7–17

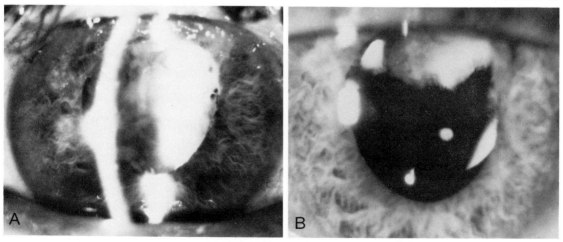

(A) Retained cortical material after ECCE with PC IOL has swollen behind the IOL and occluded the visual axis. No resorption was evident after two weeks. *(B)* "Corticolysis" resulted in liquefaction of the cortical material and clearing of the visual axis within one week.

Postoperative Care. As mentioned previously, pressure elevation and inflammation may be more pronounced than with simple capsulotomy. This result should be anticipated, and steroids and glaucoma medications should be administered as indicated.

REFERENCES

1. Aron-Rosa D, Aron JJ, Griesemann M, Thyzel R. Use of the neodymium-YAG laser to open the posterior capsule after lens implant surgery. A preliminary report. J Am Intraocul Implant Soc 6:352–4, 1980.
2. Aron-Rosa D, Griesemann JC, Aron JJ. Use of a pulsed neodymium-YAG laser (picosecond) to open the posterior lens capsule in traumatic cataract: A preliminary report. Ophthalmic Surg 12:496–9, 1981.
3. Fankhauser F, Lortscher H, Van der Zypen E. Clinical studies on high and low power laser radiation upon some structures of the anterior and posterior segments of the eye. Int Ophthalmol 5:15–32, 1982.
4. The Miami Study Group. Cystoid macular edema in aphakic and pseudophakic eyes. Am J Ophthalmol 88:45–8, 1979.
5. Jaffe NS, Luscombe SM, Clayman HM, Gass JD. A fluorescein angiographic study of cystoid macular edema. Am J Ophthalmol 92:775–7, 1981.
6. Jaffe NS, Clayman HM, Jaffe MS. Cystoid macular edema after intracapsular cataract extraction with and without an intraocular lens. Ophthalmol 89:25–9, 1982.
7. Wetzig PC, Thatcher DB, Christiansen JM. The intracapsular versus the extracapsular technique in relationship to retinal problems. Trans Am Ophthalmol Soc 77:339–47, 1979.
8. Chambliss WS. Phacoemulsification and the retina: Cystoid macular edema. Ophthalmology 86:2019–22, 1979.
9. Yannuzzi LA, Landau AN, Turtz AI. Incidence of aphakic cystoid macular edema with the use of topical indomethacin. Ophthalmology 88:947–54, 1981.
10. Kraff MC, Sanders DR, Jampol LM, Lieberman HL. Effect of primary capsulotomy with extracapsular surgery on the incidence of pseudophakic cystoid macular edema. Am J Ophthalmol 98:166–70, 1984.
11. Moses L. Cystoid macular edema and retinal detachment following cataract surgery. J Am Intraocul Implant Soc 5:326–9, 1979.
12. Sorr EM, Everett WG, Hurite FG. Incidence of fluorescein angiographic subclinical macular edema following phacoemulsification of senile cataracts. Ophthalmology 86:2013–8, 1979.
13. Hurite F, Sorr EM, Everett WG. The incidence of retinal detachment following phacoemulsification. Ophthalmology 86:2004–06, 1979.
14. Clayman HM, Jaffe NS, Light DS, Jaffe MS, Cassady JC. Intraocular lenses, axial length, and retinal detachment. Am J Ophthalmol 92:778–80, 1981.
15. Jaffe NS. Cataract Surgery and Its Complications. 3rd ed. St. Louis: C V Mosby Company, 1976, pp 576–88.
16. Binkhorst CD, Kato A, Tjan TT. Retinal accidents in pseudophakia. Intracapsular vs. extracapsular surgery. Trans Am Acad Ophthalmol Otolaryngol 81:120–7, 1976.
17. Jaffe NS, Clayman HM, Jaffe MS. Retinal detachment in myopic eyes after intracapsular and extracapsular cataract extraction. Am J Ophthalmol 97:48–52, 1984.
18. Sinskey RM, Cain W. The posterior capsule and phacoemulsification. J Am Intraocul Implant Soc 4:206–7, 1978.
19. Emery JM, Wilhelmus KR, Rosenberg S. Complications of phacoemulsification. Ophthalmology 85:141–50, 1978.
20. Wilhelmus KR, Emery JM. Posterior capsule opacification following phacoemulsification. In Emery JM, Jacobson AC (eds.). Current Concepts in Cataract Surgery: Selected Proceedings of the Sixth Biennial Cataract Surgical Congress. St. Louis: C V Mosby Company, 1980, pp 304–8.
21. McDonnell PJ, Zarbin MA, Green WR. Posterior capsule opacification in pseudophakic eyes. Ophthalmology 90:1548–53, 1983.
22. Chan RY, Emery JM, Kretzer F. Mitotic inhibitors in preventing posteror lens capsule opacification. In Emery JM, Jacobson AC (eds.). Current Concepts in Cataract Surgery: Selected Proceedings of the Seventh Biennial Cataract Surgical Congress. New York: Appleton-Century-Crofts, 1982, pp 217–24.
23. Knolle G. Office discissions of the posterior capsule (intraocular lens in situ). In Emery JM, Jacobson AC (eds.). Current Concepts in Cataract Surgery: Selected Proceedings of the Seventh Biennial Cataract Surgical Congress. New York: Appleton-Century-Crofts, 1982, pp 225–7.
24. Jaffe NS. Cataract Surgery and Its Complications. 4th ed. St. Louis: C V Mosby Company, 1981, pp 167–9.
25. Lindstrom RL, Harris WS. Management of the posterior capsule following posterior chamber lens implantation. J Am Intraocul Implant Soc 6:255–8, 1980.

26. Jaffe NS. Cystoid macular edema with intracapsular and extracapsular cataract extraction. *In* Emery JM, Jacobson AC (eds). Current Concepts in Cataract Surgery: Selected Proceedings of the Seventh Biennial Cataract Surgical Congress. New York: Appleton-Century-Crofts, 1982, pp 231–2.
27. Livernois R, Sinskey RM. Complications of late capsulotomy. J Am Intraocul Implant Soc 7:242–3, 1981.
28. McPherson AR, O'Malley RE, Bravo J. Retinal detachment following late posterior capsulotomy. Am J Ophthalmol 95:593–7, 1983.
29. Terry AC, Stark WJ, Maumenee AE, Fagadau W. Neodymium-YAG laser for posterior capsulotomy. Am J Ophthalmol 96:716–20, 1983.
30. Fastenberg DM, Schwartz PL, Lin HZ. Retinal detachment following neodymium-YAG laser capsulotomy. Am J Ophthalmol 97:288–91, 1984.
31. Parker WT, Clorfeine GS, Stocklin RD. Marked intraocular pressure rise following Nd-YAG laser capsulotomy. Ophthalmic Surg 15:103–4, 1984.
32. Keates RH, Steinert RF, Puliafito CA, Maxwell SK. Long-term follow-up of Nd-YAG laser posterior capsulotomy. J Am Intraocul Implant Soc 10:164–8, 1984.
33. Channell MM, Beckman H. Intraocular pressure changes after Neodymium-YAG laser posterior capsulotomy. Arch Ophthalmol 102:1024–6, 1984.
34. Richter CU, Arzeno G, Pappas H, Steinert RF, Puliafito CA, Epstein DL. Acute changes in intraocular pressure and tonography after Nd-YAG laser capsulomy. (In preparation.)
35. Epstein DL, Jedziniak JA, Grant WM. Obstruction of aqueous outflow by lens particles and by heavy molecular-weight soluble lens proteins. Invest Ophthalmol Vis Sci 17:272–7, 1978.
36. Faulkner W. Laser interferometric prediction of postoperative visual acuity in patients with cataracts. Am J Ophthalmol 95:626–36, 1983.
37. Riggins J, Pedrotti LS, Keates RH. Evaluation of the neodymium-YAG laser for treatment of ocular opacities. Ophthalmic Surg 14:675–82, 1983.
38. Nadler DL, Jaffe NS, Clayman HM, Jaffe MS, Luscombe SM. Glare disability in eyes with intraocular lenses. Am J Ophthalmol 97:43–7, 1984.
39. Vine AK. Ocular hypertension following Nd-YAG laser capsulotomy: A potentially blinding complication. Ophthalmic Surg 15:283–4, 1984.
40. Ruderman JM, Mitchell PG, Kraff M. Pupillary bock following Nd-YAG capsulotomy. Ophthalmic Surg 14:418–9, 1983.
41. Shrader CE, Belcher CD III, Thomas JV, Simmons RJ. Acute glaucoma following Nd-YAG laser membranotomy. Ophthalmic Surg 14:1015–6, 1983.
42. Fankhauser F, Roussel P, Steffen J, Van der Zypen E, Chrenkova A. Clinical studies on the efficiency of high power laser radiation upon some structures of the anterior segment of the eye. Int Ophthalmol 3:129–39, 1981.

8

LASER-IOL DAMAGE AND LASER-DESIGN IOLs

LASER-IOL DAMAGE STUDIES

High-irradiance laser pulses from Q-switched and mode-locked lasers may mark an intraocular lens (IOL). The physics of damage to glass and polymethylmethacrylate (PMMA) are reviewed in Chapter 3. Because irregularities and imperfections may serve as starting points for laser damage, manufacturing techniques that lead to excellent surface finishing and minimize internal microvoids, irregularities, and imperfections should reduce the tendency for IOL damage.

Clinically, PMMA damage takes the form of small surface pits and internal cracks, usually less than 0.5 mm in length, that pass obliquely at a 45-degree angle through the body of the lens. The physical basis for this orientation is explained on p. 33. These cracks appear black against a red reflex and have been coined "flying saucers." Occasionally, a vapor bubble may be seen issuing from the crack within a second after the laser shot. A large pit and a crack are seen against the red reflex in Figure 8–1.

Edge-to-edge full-thickness cracks may occur with glass IOLs (Fig. 8–2), whereas this phenomenon has never been reported with a PMMA IOL.

Representative scanning electron micrographs (SEMs) of laser-induced IOL damage are shown in Figures 8–3 through 8–7.

Johnson, Kratz, and Olson have performed extensive studies on the effect of Nd-YAG laser damage on the Air Force target resolution capability of a variety of commercial IOLs.* Despite extensive damage greatly exceeding that in typical clinical experience, all lenses retained resolving power in excess of the equivalent of 20/10 vision.

Although a laser-damaged IOL continues to provide excellent target resolution under standard conditions, it is reasonable to expect that this type of damage could result in glare. There is no generally agreed upon laboratory test for glare. However, laser-damaged IOLs were evaluated using the photographic system described in Chapter 7. A normal lens was compared with a lens having ten small central pits and with a lens having ten central cracks (Fig. 8–8). All three lenses showed comparable clarity when the Snellen chart was

*Johnson SH 1984: personal communication.

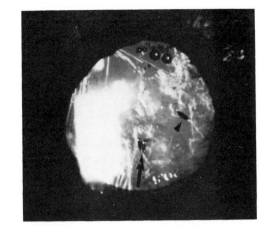

FIGURE 8–1

Red reflex view shows a large pit *(arrow)* and a crack *(arrowhead)* in a posterior chamber IOL after Nd-YAG laser capsulotomy.

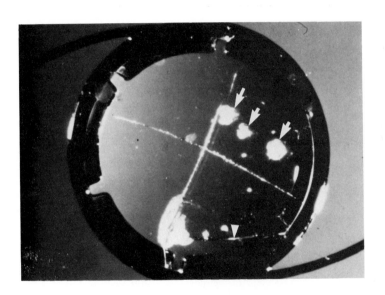

FIGURE 8–2

Multiple large surface pits *(arrows)* and an edge-to-edge crack *(arrowhead)* were created experimentally by 4-mJ Q-switched pulses fired into a glass IOL divided into quadrants. (Courtesy of Stephen H. Johnson.)

FIGURE 8–3

Scanning election micrograph of a surface pit and cracking created by a 2-mJ laser pulse on the posterior surface of a glass IOL. Original magnification 220×. (Courtesy of Steven H. Johnson.)

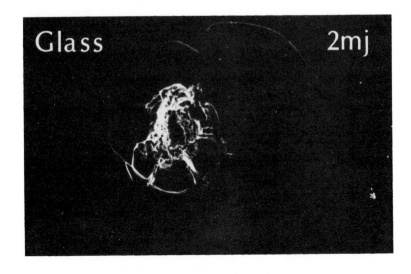

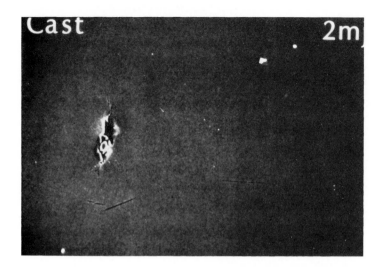

FIGURE 8–4

Scanning election micrograph of a small surface pit created by a 2-mJ pulse on the posterior surface of a cast-molded IOL. Original magnification 220×. (Courtesy of Steven H. Johnson.)

FIGURE 8–5

Scanning election micrograph of a large surface pit created by a 2-mJ pulse on the posterior surface of a compression-molded IOL. Note the fragments that have settled on adjacent IOL surfaces. Original magnification 220×. (Courtesy of Stephen H. Johnson.)

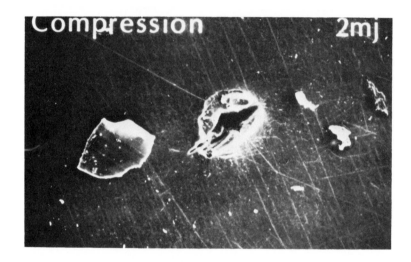

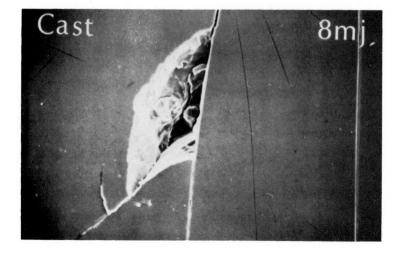

FIGURE 8–6

More extensive pitting and cracking occurs with higher energy, as shown in this scanning electron micrograph of a cast-molded lens struck on its posterior surface by an 8-mJ pulse. Comparison should be made with the effect of a 2-mJ pulse, as shown in Figure 8–4. Original magnification 220×. (Courtesy of Stephen H. Johnson.)

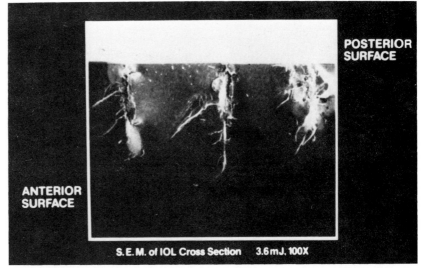

FIGURE 8–7

Scanning election micrograph of a section through cracks caused by 3.6-mJ pulses on the posterior surface of a lathe-cut IOL. Original magnification 100×. (Courtesy of Thomas J. Westman.)

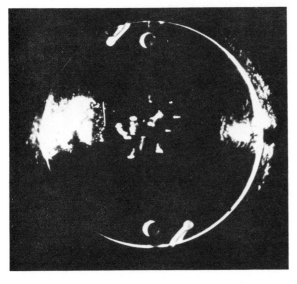

FIGURE 8–8

Side-illuminated photograph of an IOL with ten central cracks used in a photographic glare study.

FIGURE 8–9

Glare caused by laser-induced cracks in the IOL shown in Figure 8–8 *(above)*. Comparison should be made with the lack of glare in the control normal lens in Figure 7–13*J*.

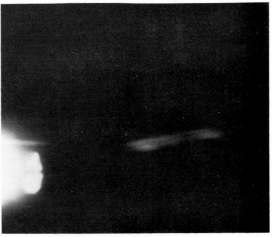

99

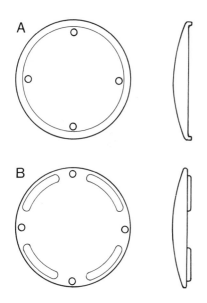

FIGURE 8–10

(A) A 360-degree peripheral ring on the posterior IOL surface, originally intended to prevent capsular opacification, can facilitate laser capsulotomy without marking the lens by separating the posterior capsule from the IOL. *(B)* Busses on the posterior IOL surface represent a partial ring.

FIGURE 8–11

A concave posterior surface gives a central separation from the capsule, which diminishes toward the periphery.

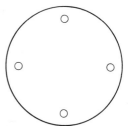
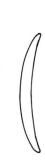

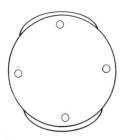
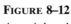

FIGURE 8–12

A peripheral "tab" lens, with the tabs oriented along the axis of the haptics, offers uniform separation of lens and capsule without thickening of the edge or reduction of the useful optical zone.

TABLE 8–1. PRINCIPLES OF THE OPTIMAL LASER-DESIGN IOL

1. Adequate separation is obtained (0.2 mm or more).
2. Separation is maintained throughout the optical zone.
3. The optical zone is not reduced.
4. Capsule pressure should tend to flatten wrinkles along the haptic axis.
5. Edge thickness is not increased.
6. Wound and pupillary size requirements are unchanged.
7. The IOL edge allows use of conventional insertion forceps and techniques without instability or risk of crush damage.
8. There is little or no weight increase.

photographed, as was expected on the basis of the Air Force target resolution studies.

When an automobile headlight was used as a source of glare, neither the normal lens nor the lens with ten small pits showed detectable glare. The lens with cracks, however, exhibited considerable glare in certain positions (Fig. 8–9).

In conclusion, YAG laser IOL marks are much less visually debilitating than a capsular opacity. Marks may cause glare, however, and their avoidance is desirable.

LASER-DESIGN IOLs

With accurate focusing, IOL marks generally can be avoided if the IOL is adequately separated from the capsule. No one separation distance is precisely adequate in all situations. However, early clinical experience and unpublished studies* have indicated that a separation of at least 0.2 mm is adequate in most situations.

Separation of the posterior capsule from the IOL can be achieved in three general ways. The first is by the use of a full ring or a series of busses placed around the edge of the posterior IOL optic, as shown in Figure 8–10. Kenneth Hoffer originated the ring lens in an effort to create a pressure barrier to prevent the migration of epithelial cells across the posterior capsule. The validity of this concept has not been generally accepted, but the lens does provide a space between IOL and capsule to allow laser capsulotomy when opacification does occur.

A second approach is to use an IOL with a concave posterior surface (Fig. 8–11). This lens does not thicken the edge or reduce the optical zone. The lens must have a greater anterior vault to obtain the same refractive power. The specified separation is present only at the center and diminishes progressively with movement toward the periphery of the optic.

The third approach is a protrusion or a "tab" extending from the optic outward and posteriorly (Fig. 8–12). If the tab is oriented along the axis of the haptics, it does not increase insertion width or edge thickness or reduce the optical zone. The tab provides uniform separation throughout most of its width and may tend to flatten wrinkles. No 360-degree barrier effect is provided.

Choice of a laser-design IOL is a matter of clinical preference. The principles of a theoretically optimal laser-design IOL are given in Table 8–1.

---

*Myers WD 1984: personal communication.

9

PHOTODISRUPTION OF THE IRIS: IRIDECTOMY, COREOPLASTY, SYNECHIALYSIS

PHAKIC IRIDECTOMY

The argon laser is capable of creating a peripheral iridectomy in most patients by thermal coagulation, vaporization, and necrosis.[1, 2] Failure to achieve a full-thickness opening occasionally occurs, particularly in blue, gray, or thick dark brown irides. In lightly pigmented irides, such as blue or gray ones, argon blue-green or pure green light is poorly absorbed by the iris stroma. Adequate light absorption to achieve an opening depends on heating the underlying melanotic pigment epithelium. If perforation is not rapidly obtained before the pigment epithelium is dispersed, further attempts at perforation at that site become futile. Thick brown irides may build up a char that impedes further penetration.

Complications of argon laser iridectomy include corneal burns, local lenticular opacity, retinal burns, transient elevation of intraocular pressure, and closure of an initially patent iridectomy.

Photodisruption, unlike photocoagulation, does not depend on the pigmentation of the target. The Nd-YAG laser offers the alternative of opening the iris by cutting, rather than burning, and is particularly attractive for cases in which argon iridectomy has been attempted unsuccessfully. In phakic patients, however, the proximity of the underlying lens capsule raises concern for inadvertent rupture of the capsule with resultant cataract formation.

Fankhauser and coworkers were the first to use Q-switched Nd-YAG laser photodisruption for iridectomy.[3, 4] They had 100 per cent success in achieving a patent iridectomy in their first 85 patients. Late closure of the iridectomy was not mentioned. Opacification of the underlying anterior lens capsule for 1 to 2 mm was observed in some patients; the opacities cleared and no cataract formation was seen. Bleeding was rare and quickly resorbed. Haze of the overlying cornea that cleared in several days also occurred occasionally. Schwartz believes that the complications of Nd-YAG iridectomy are similar to those of argon iridectomy but generally less severe.[1] In particular, a transient

TABLE 9–1. COMPLICATIONS OF Nd-YAG LASER IRIDECTOMY

1. Iritis
2. Pigment dispersion
3. Hemorrhage
4. Transient intraocular pressure elevation
5. Lens opacities
6. Rupture of anterior lens capsule
7. Localized corneal edema or scar
8. Failure to obtain patent iridectomy
9. Late closure of iridectomy
10. Transient pain and blurred vision

self-limited trickling hemorrhage was found in 25 per cent of YAG cases, whereas this is never seen in coagulation after argon laser treatment. Other complications were of the same or lesser severity than with argon lasers. Both techniques showed a small elevation of intraocular pressure one hour after treatment that had resolved by three hours. Lens opacities or capsule rupture were not seen. Table 9–1 lists reported complications and the more likely potential complications.

The authors' early results with Nd-YAG laser phakic iridectomy have been favorable. Full-thickness iridectomy is achieved more quickly and reliably with the Nd-YAG laser than with the argon laser. Penetration usually occurs with a single shot. Unlike cutting through the iris sphincter, in which bleeding is the rule (see later discussion of coreoplasty), peripheral iridectomy rarely involves bleeding. Inflammation and discomfort are minimal. Lens capsule damage has not yet been observed. The overlying cornea remains clear.

Experimental studies have supported the efficacy and safety of YAG laser iridectomy when it is properly performed. Of potential interest is the tendency of the shock wave of the YAG pulse to clear a zone of pigment epithelium larger than the iridectomy opening itself.[5–7] Clinical studies comparing long-term results with argon and YAG laser iridectomies are necessary to determine whether one technique has a reduced likelihood of late closure related to proliferation of pigment epithelium.

Experimental iridectomies in pigmented rabbits were performed with the Q-switched Nd-YAG laser through iris in direct apposition to the paracentral lens to assess potential lens injury.[7] Focal deposition of pigment epithelium on the lens capsule was found frequently. A hazy white capsular opacity appearing within minutes to hours and resolving within two weeks was seen underlying iridectomies conducted at 4 to 6 mJ. At high pulse energies of 12 mJ or more, granular white permanent focal lens opacities were created that were similar in appearance to argon-laser–induced opacities. These opacities did not progress or resolve in up to 30 days. A dye study indicated that the lens capsule remained intact in all cases. An experimental shock-wave–induced focal lens opacity, of the transient type, is shown in Figure 9–1.

Richardson and coworkers have also demonstrated in experimental Q-switched Nd-YAG laser iridectomy that shock-wave damage to trabecular and corneal endothelium can occur to tissues within approximately 1 mm of the target, as shown in Figure 9–2. This finding is consistent with the clinical observation of occasional transient corneal opacity overlying Q-switched iridectomies. The possible long-term clinical significance is unknown.

TECHNIQUE FOR PHAKIC IRIDECTOMY

Preparation of the Patient. The general preparation for YAG laser treatment, including obtaining patient informed consent, is outlined in Chapter 7. Particular preparation for peripheral iridectomy includes administration of

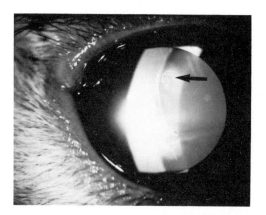

FIGURE 9–1

Focal anterior lens opacity induced experimentally by a single 6-mJ Q-switched pulse applied 1 to 2 mm anterior to the lens capsule of a rabbit *(arrow)*. The vertically oriented lens suture line is unrelated.

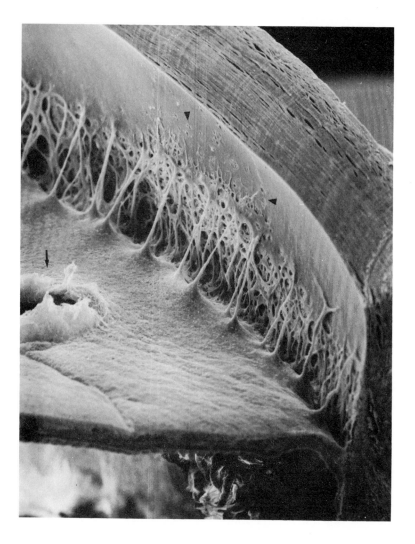

FIGURE 9–2

Scanning electron micrograph of an experimental Q-switched Nd-YAG laser iridectomy made by five shots at 5 mJ in an owl monkey eye *(arrow)* using a nonfundamental mode laser. Damage to adjacent trabecular and corneal endothelium is apparent *(arrowheads)*. The pressure wave and tissue debris presumably shear off the cells. Original magnification 40×. (Courtesy of Thomas Richardson.)

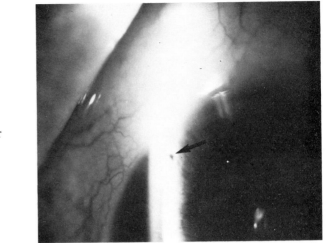

FIGURE 9–3

Phakic peripheral iridectomy performed by a single 4 mJ fumdamental mode Nd-YAG laser shot (*arrow*).

miotics. The application of pilocarpine 4 per cent every 15 minutes beginning two hours before the procedure greatly facilitates the iridectomy by stretching the iris. Topical anesthetic drops are given at the time of treatment.

Procedure. The Abraham lens with a peripheral 66 diopter button lens is applied, and a basal site is selected. The peripheral crystalline lens is not in direct apposition to the basal iris, so that an extra margin of safety is provided. A thin area such as a crypt is preferable to facilitate penetration and avoid bleeding. The usual energy setting is 4 to 8 mJ. The laser is carefully aimed and fired. A full-thickness opening in one shot is desirable, although up to four shots are commonly needed. Once an opening is obtained, or if it is unclear whether an opening is patent, it is inadvisable to continue with a "chipping" technique, which exposes the lens capsule to the laser pulse if any unexpected movement of the eye occurs. Use of a burst mode, particularly one longer than several pulses, also potentially exposes the underlying lens capsule to injury if the iris opening is obtained before the burst is completed. Figure 9–3 shows a phakic Q-switched Nd-YAG laser iridectomy.

Postoperative Care. Investigational protocols, when applicable, must be followed. In particular, pressure, inflammation, bleeding, and lens clarity should be monitored.

Administration of a strong topical steroid such as prednisolone 1 per cent or dexamethasone 0.1 per cent is begun immediately with application four times a day. The importance of postlaser dilation or miosis has not been demonstrated. In the presence of clinically significant bleeding or inflammation, if the iridectomy is definitely patent, intermittent short-term dilation is advisable to avoid synechia.

APHAKIC AND PSEUDOPHAKIC IRIDECTOMY AND ANTERIOR HYALOID VITREOLYSIS

Acute angle closure glaucoma in aphakia and pseudophakia may take several forms, as outlined in Table 9–2.[8, 9] Corneal edema and haze, anterior chamber reaction, and iris congestion may make argon laser iridectomy impossible. Even when a patent opening is created, an argon laser iridectomy may not relieve the glaucoma because of the role of the vitreous. In the authors' opinion the YAG laser can better treat these conditions, and this is the treatment of first choice.[10] The success of the Nd-YAG laser "anterior hyaloidectomy" in curing ciliovitreal block glaucoma, in which surgical and argon iridectomies have failed, demonstrates the pathophysiologic role of the anterior hyaloid face and represents a major advance in treatment.

TABLE 9–2. ACUTE APHAKIC AND PSEUDOPHAKIC GLAUCOMA

Pupillary block (iridovitreal block)
    Absent, imperforate, or secluded peripheral iridectomies
    Inflammatory adhesion of intact hyaloid face to iris
    Anterior chamber hemorrhage and exudate
Aphakic malignant glaucoma (ciliovitreal block)
    Posterior diversion of aqueous

Figure 9–4 illustrates a case of pupillary block in a patient who had vitrectomy and antibiotic therapy for endophthalmitis after extracapsular cataract extraction with an anterior chamber IOL. The surgical iridectomies closed postoperatively, but the argon laser succeeded in relieving the resultant iris bombé. Within weeks the argon laser iridectomies closed, and the iris bombé recurred with a pressure of 50 mm Hg. The Nd-YAG laser at 4 mJ readily created several new iridectomies with relief of the iris bombé and pressure elevation. The pupillary membrane also was cleared by the Nd-YAG laser.

An uncomplicated intracapsular cataract extraction with an anterior chamber (AC) IOL was performed on a patient, as illustrated in Figure 9–5. On the first postoperative day a shallow chamber and elevated pressure were found. A large patent surgical iridectomy was visible, and the pupil was dilated beyond the IOL optic without relief. Argon laser iridectomies also failed to provide relief. The anterior hyaloid face was intact. The Nd-YAG laser was fired through the argon iridectomies to provide immediate deepening of the chamber and resolution of the glaucoma. The subsequent postoperative course was unremarkable.

The role of the hyaloid face in aphakic malignant glaucoma is further illustrated by the case shown in Color Plates *I*C and *D*. Three months after complicated cataract extraction and subsequent IOL removal in a patient who had had a large superior sector iridectomy, the chamber became shallow and the pressure rose to 34 mm Hg over several days with the onset of deep pain. A thin intact hyaloid face was present. The patient was treated with the YAG laser, which was focused and fired at 3 mJ on the hyaloid face through mild corneal edema and with less than 1 mm of anterior chamber depth. The chamber deepened immediately.

FIGURE 9–4

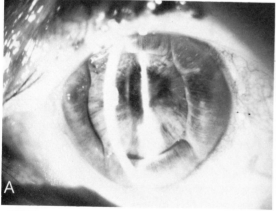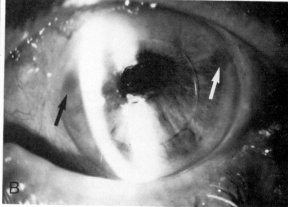

(A) Recurrent pseudophakic pupillary block with iris bombé after endophthalmitis and closure of argon laser iridectomy. *(B)* The Nd-YAG laser at 4 mJ readily created several iridectomies *(arrows)* with permanent relief of the iris bombé. A pupillary membranectomy was also performed.

FIGURE 9–5

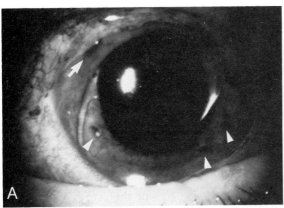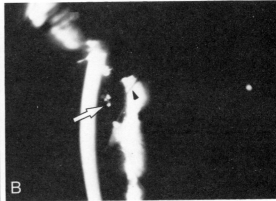

(A) One day after intracapsular cataract extraction with an anterior chamber IOL, elevated pressure and a shallow chamber were found. The anterior hyaloid membrane was intact. The pupil had dilated beyond the optic inferiorly, and the iris had prolapsed over the superior optic. Patent argon iridectomies *(arrowheads)* provided no relief. A large basal surgical iridectomy was present *(arrow)*. *(B)* After the YAG laser had been fired through the argon laser iridectomies, the chamber immediately deepened. Loose vitreous humor could be seen in the anterior chamber *(arrow)*. The iris returned to proper position behind the optic *(arrowhead)*. (Reproduced from Epstein DL, Steinert RF, Puliafito CA. Neodymium-YAG laser therapy to the anterior hyaloid in aphakic malignant (ciliovitreal block) glaucoma. Am J Ophthalmol 98:137–43, 1984. With permission from Ophthalmic Publishing Co.)

The Nd-YAG laser can also successfully forestall more invasive procedures in some cases. The first day after intracapsular cataract extraction with an anterior chamber IOL, the case in Color Plate I*E* was found to have a hemorrhage located inferiorly that covered the IOL optic. The superior iris was in apposition to the cornea. Intraocular pressure was 26 mm Hg. The patient was scheduled for emergency IOL removal and anterior vitrectomy when the YAG laser was considered. Nd-YAG laser iridectomies made superiorly resulted in immediate chamber deepening, as shown in Color Plate I*F*. The condition of the eye normalized, and the hemorrhage slowly cleared. Ultimately vision recovered to 20/70.

TECHNIQUE FOR APHAKIC AND PSEUDOPHAKIC IRIDECTOMY AND ANTERIOR HYALOID VITREOLYSIS

Preparation of the Patient. The usual protocol including informed consent is followed (see Chapter 7).

Procedure. Four to 8 mJ is usually adequate to perforate the iris in one shot. Corneal edema or anterior chamber reaction may necessitate higher energy to obtain the same cutting power. At least three iridectomies should be made to ensure full relief of aqueous entrapment, which may be localized into sectors, and to increase the chance of maintaining at least one long-term patent iridectomy. Iridectomies tend to shrink as bombé is relieved and the iris falls back. Inflammation also may close iridectomies subsequently.

If the chamber is markedly shallow or flat, the haptic of an anterior chamber pseudophakos, when present, usually provides a small area of clearance from the cornea. The first shots can be made immediately adjacent to such a haptic insertion to avoid corneal damage.

After the iridectomy has been completed or when a patent basal iridectomy is already present, the YAG laser should be fired into the anterior vitreous through the iridectomy or the pupil. This procedure ruptures the hyaloid face and relieves any malignant glaucoma caused by the intact hyaloid face.

Postoperative Care. Intensive topical steroid therapy (prednisolone 1 per cent, dexamethasone 0.1 per cent) is used at least four times per day and more often as inflammation requires. Inflammation and a tendency for synechia formation require cycloplegia and mydriasis. Intraocular pressure must be monitored and treated appropriately.

COREOPLASTY

The Nd-YAG laser can cut through iris stroma or the pupillary sphincter to open an occluded visual axis. Indications for coreoplasty are pupillary enlargement for vision or improvement of the fundus view for examination and treatment. Synechialysis can also affect pupillary configuration, as is discussed in the next section.

Figure 9–6 (*A* to *C*) illustrates a case in which the pupil became drawn upward after intracapsular cataract extraction. The upper lid covered the pupil. When the lid was elevated, vision was limited to the level of counting fingers. The Nd-YAG laser cut through the sphincter with only a localized self-limited trickling hemorrhage. Vision improved to 20/70 and was limited only by pre-existing maculopathy.

Color Plate I*B* shows a similar result in a patient with long-term poor vision caused by an eccentric pupil after cataract wound rupture. Optical iridectomy improved vision to 20/40.

The case shown in Figure 9–7 involved a corneal laceration with traumatic cataract. After healing, synechia to the posterior capsule drew the pupil inferiorly and under the overlying corneal scar. An opaque posterior capsule

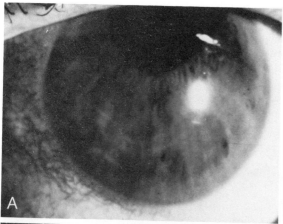
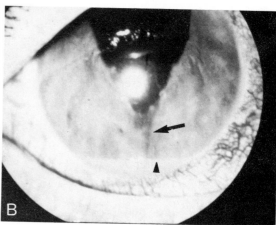
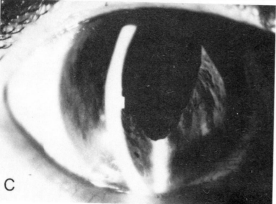

FIGURE 9–6

(A) Updrawn pupil after intracapsular cataract extraction. *(B)* Immediately after sphincterotomy, a candle-wax–like trickle of blood was seen clotted at the inferior margin of the sphincterotomy *(arrow)*. A light reflection from the lid margin gave an appearance similar to hypopyon *(arrowhead)*, but no gross hemorrhage or inflammation occurred. *(C)* One week later, the clot had cleared, and the central cornea was in the optical axis.

FIGURE 9–7

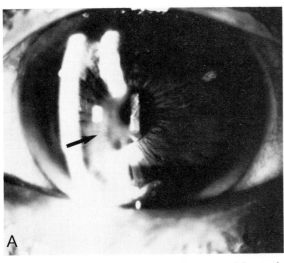
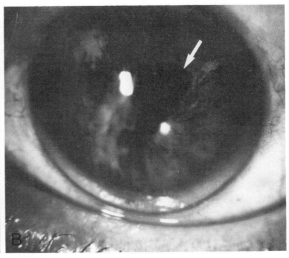

(A) A penetrating corneal laceration *(arrow)* and a traumatic cataract left the patient with a hazy capsule and a pupil bound by synechiae to the area under the scar and the adjacent optically irregular cornea. (B) Sphincterotomy enlarged the pupil *(arrow)* so that it moved away from the scar into clear cornea. The posterior capsule was also opened. Vision improved from 20/80 to 20/40.

was also present. The Nd-YAG laser was used to perform a sphincterotomy, enlarging the pupil toward the normal clear cornea. Posterior capsulotomy was also performed. Vision improved from 20/80 to 20/40.

In Figure 9–8, multiple small sphincterotomies along with lysis of synechia to the anterior hyaloid face were used to improve pupillary dilation to facilitate peripheral panretinal photocoagulation for diabetic retinopathy.

TECHNIQUE FOR COREOPLASTY

Preparation of the Patient. The general preparation for YAG laser treatment, including obtaining the patient's informed consent, is outlined in

FIGURE 9–8

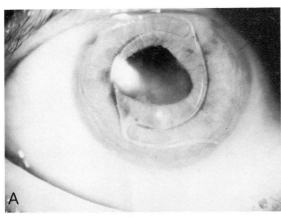
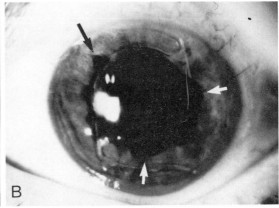

(A) After intensive instillation of cycloplegics and mydriatics, pupillary dilation was inadequate to allow a satisfactory view of the peripheral retina for panretinal argon laser photocoagulation for proliferative diabetic retinopathy. (B) Synechia to the anterior hyaloid face were lysed, and three small sphincterotomies *(arrows)* were made to allow wider pupillary dilation.

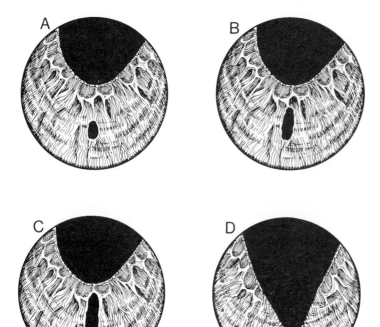

FIGURE 9–9

Technique for Nd-YAG laser sphincterotomy. *(A)* The treatment is begun in the peripheral iris stroma. *(B, C)* Progressive cutting is made toward the iris sphincter. *(D)* The sphincter is cut last so that bleeding is minimized for as long as possible to increase the chance of completing the treatment in one session.

Chapter 7. Information regarding the presence of bleeding abnormalities must be specifically elicited in taking the history, since clotting abnormalities increase the risk of a large hyphema.

In the authors' experience, preparatory thermal iris photocoagulation, whether by argon or long-pulse thermal YAG laser, has not been necessary or helpful for most cases. Very heavy and extensive iris coagulation is necessary to prevent bleeding when the pulsed YAG laser is subsequently used. The pressure wave after optical breakdown radiates over several millimeters with enough shearing force to cause capillary oozing, and thus it is difficult to eliminate bleeding without widespread intense preparatory coagulation. An exception to this principle is a visible blood vessel whose path cannot be avoided; it would be folly to cut such a vessel with the YAG laser without thorough prior photocoagulation. Patients in whom preparatory laser coagulation has been performed generally state that the photocoagulation is more painful than the photodisruption.

Procedure. Six to 10 mJ is the usual setting. Numerous shots are required to cut across 3 to 5 mm of sphincter and stroma.

The sphincter is the toughest region to cut and, with the minor arterial circle, the most prone to hemorrhage. If the surgeon starts at the pupil and cuts across the sphincter first, gross hemorrhage and free red cells and fibrin in the anterior chamber may prevent completion of the treatment in one session. To avoid significant hemorrhage until nearly the end of the session the treatment should begin in the peripheral iris stroma and progress toward the sphincter and pupil. Figure 9–9 illustrates a sequential sphincterotomy.

If bleeding begins without clotting and does not cease rapidly, pressure should be applied to the globe through a contact lens, if one is being used, or by a finger through the lids or a cotton swab applied to the globe. Pressure adequate to stop the bleeding is maintained for several minutes until effective iris vessel coagulation has time to occur.

Postoperative Care. A strong steroid (prednisolone 1 per cent or dexamethasone 0.1 per cent) is given topically four times daily initially, with the dosage tapered as inflammation subsides. Cycloplegia is usually unnecessary. Intraocular pressure elevation should be monitored and treated appropriately.

SYNECHIALYSIS

Localized synechiae with associated pigment may be broken by photocoagulation with the argon laser. Generally, however, the Nd-YAG laser is more successful than the argon laser in synechialysis because pigmentation of the target is not required and forceful rupture of adhesions can be made.

An inflammatory band had hemisected the pupil of the patient in Figure 9–10, who was referred for posterior capsulotomy a year after extracapsular cataract extraction with a posterior chamber IOL. The pupillary distortion was unesthetic but visually insignificant. After completion of the capsulotomy, the Nd-YAG laser beam was repeatedly shot at the fibrous band near the superior sphincter. The band frayed like a rope and finally broke under tension. The pupil rounded immediately. The underlying IOL was undamaged (see also the case in Fig. 11–1), indicating that the shock wave alone does not primarily damage an IOL, but rather that IOL marks are caused by optical breakdown, plasma formation, and stimulated Brillouin scattering when damage occurs within the lens (see Chapter 3, pp. 32–34). Since these processes tend to grow in an anterior direction and are relatively shielded posteriorly, the IOL is undamaged by optical breakdown occurring anterior to the IOL. This is the converse of the clinical problem of marking the posterior surface of an IOL adjacent to a posterior capsule.

Synechiae can displace a posterior chamber IOL. One month after uneventful extracapsular cataract extraction with a posterior chamber IOL, on a routine follow-up examination a patient was found to have inferior iris capture of the IOL. Strong dilation revealed pigmented synechia to the posterior capsule (Fig. 9–11). The argon laser was available and was used to break the synechia but the IOL capture persisted. Examination then disclosed that relatively unpigmented synechiae had formed at the points of haptic insertion into this Sinskey-style lens, which had been dialed into a horizontal position.

FIGURE 9–10

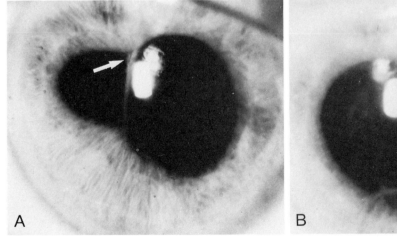

A   B

(A) A synechial band lying on the anterior surface of a posterior chamber IOL runs across the pupil, dividing it. With repeated shots the Nd-YAG laser cut the band at the point indicated by the arrow. *(B)* After the band had been cut, it retracted and curled inferiorly, and the pupil became more round. There was no damage to the underlying IOL.

FIGURE 9–11

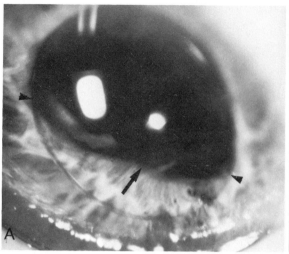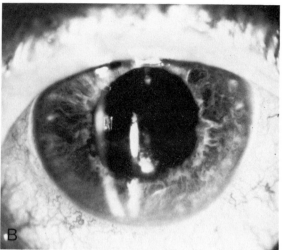

(A) Inferior iris capture of a posterior chamber IOL, with pigmented synechiae to the posterior capsule visible after dilation *(arrow)*. Significant nonpigmented synechiae were also present at the 3 and 9 o'clock positions at the haptic insertions into the optic *(arrowheads) (B),* Lysing of the inferior synechiae alone was inadequate. The IOL fell back into place only when the synechiae around the haptic insertions were broken.

The YAG laser at 6 mJ readily broke these synechiae. When the last synechia was released, the IOL relaxed back into position behind the iris.

Synechiae can form around anterior chamber IOL footplates. This condition may lead to pupillary distortion in the absence of tuck. In Figure 9–12*A* the pupil is seen to be eccentric. The patient complained bitterly of edge glare. Gonioscopy revealed synechia in association with the IOL footplates and haptic struts (Figure 9–12*B*). Synechialysis through a gonioscopy lens was carried out, requiring four sessions before the pupil moved behind the edge of the IOL and the symptoms were relieved (Figure 9–12*D*). A vessel in the inflamed peripheral iris bled after the first treatment, causing the formation of an eccentric clot. The clot disappeared over the course of one week (Figure 9–12*C*).

TECHNIQUE FOR SYNECHIALYSIS

Preparation of the Patient. General preparation of the patient, including informed consent, is discussed in Chapter 7. The patient is told beforehand that multiple sessions are often necessary for complete synechialysis. Prelaser miosis or mydriasis may help by stretching a synechia, which improves both visualization of the abnormality and the pressure wave cutting action of the laser.

Procedure. Generally the laser is set between 4 and 10 mJ, depending on the strength of the synechia to be lysed. When the abnormality can be directly visualized, the laser is aimed accordingly. Often, however, a gonioscopy lens is necessary to treat synechiae near the limbus and, of course, in the angle. Energy losses and optical aberrations often require higher laser energy settings with a gonioscopy lens in order to achieve the irradiance necessary to cut a synechia. The surgeon must titrate the energy upward until the desired effect is achieved. The gonioscopy lens and slit lamp positions must also be aligned so that the mirror captures the full laser beam and laser beam distortions caused by oblique incidence are minimized.

FIGURE 9–12

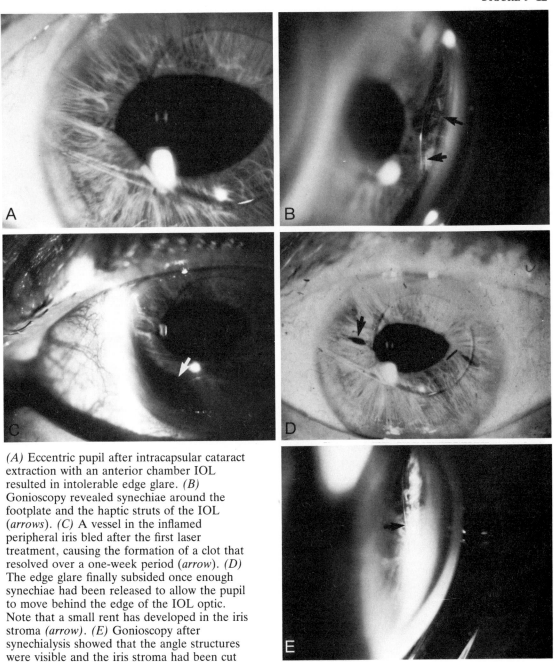

(A) Eccentric pupil after intracapsular cataract extraction with an anterior chamber IOL resulted in intolerable edge glare. (B) Gonioscopy revealed synechiae around the footplate and the haptic struts of the IOL (arrows). (C) A vessel in the inflamed peripheral iris bled after the first laser treatment, causing the formation of a clot that resolved over a one-week period (arrow). (D) The edge glare finally subsided once enough synechiae had been released to allow the pupil to move behind the edge of the IOL optic. Note that a small rent has developed in the iris stroma (arrow). (E) Gonioscopy after synechialysis showed that the angle structures were visible and the iris stroma had been cut away from the haptic strut, which runs between the two footplates (arrow).

Postoperative Care. Strong topical steroids (prednisolone 1 per cent, dexamethasone 0.1 per cent) are used initially at least four times daily and more often if severe inflammation occurs. If there is any tendency for formation of new synechiae the pupil should be moved with intermittent administration of short-acting cycloplegics and mydriatics. Intraocular pressure should be measured and appropriate treatment (using timolol or carbonic anhydrase inhibitors) should be begun when indicated.

REFERENCES

1. Schwartz L. Laser iridectomy. *In* Schwartz L, Spaeth G, Brown G. Laser Therapy of the Anterior Segment: A Practical Approach. Thorofare, NJ: Charles Slack Inc., 1984, pp 29–58.
2. Belcher CD III. Laser iridectomy. *In* Belcher CD III, Thomas JV, Simmons RJ (eds.). Photocoagulation in Glaucoma and Anterior Segment Disease. Baltimore: Williams & Wilkins, 1984, pp 87–110.
3. Fankhauser F, Roussel P, Steffen J, Van der Zypen E, Chrenkova A. Clinical studies on the efficiency of high power laser radiation upon some structures of the anterior segment of the eye. Int Ophthalmol 3:129–39, 1981.
4. Fankhauser F. The Q-switched laser: Principles and clinical results. *In* Trokel SL (ed.). YAG Laser Ophthalmic Microsurgery. Norwalk, CT: Appleton-Century-Crofts, 1983, pp 101–46.
5. Van der Zypen E, Fankhauser F, Bebie H. On the effects of different laser sources upon the iris of the pigmented rabbit. Int Ophthalmol 1:30–48, 1978.
6. Van der Zypen E, Bebie H, Fankhauser F. Morphological studies about the efficiency of laser burns on the structure of the angle of the anterior chamber. Invest Ophthalmol Vis Sci 1:109–26, 1979.
7. Latina MA, Puliafito CA, Steinert RF, Epstein DL. Experimental iridotomy with the Q-switched neodymium-YAG laser. Arch Ophthalmol 102:1211–3, 1984.
8. Shaffer RN. The role of vitreous detachment in aphakic and malignant glaucoma. Trans Am Acad Ophthalmol Otolaryngol 58:217–31, 1954.
9. Shaffer RN. A suggested anatomic classification to define the pupillary block glaucomas. Invest Ophthalmol 12:540–2, 1973.
10. Epstein DL, Steinert RF, Puliafito CA. Neodymium-YAG laser therapy to the anterior hyaloid in aphakic malignant (ciliovitreal block) glaucoma. Am J Ophthalmol 98:137–43, 1984.

10

ANTERIOR VITREOLYSIS AND CYSTOID MACULAR EDEMA

Vitreous strands and bands to the wound may cause eccentric pupils and can be associated with cystoid macular edema (Irvine-Gass CME).[1, 2] Iliff first reported visual improvement after surgical section of such vitreous bands to the wound.[3] He coined the term *vitreous-tug syndrome,* although no evidence was given that tugging on the vitreous body was in fact present or responsible for the visual loss.

Katzen, Fleischman, and Trokel first reported the use of the Nd-YAG laser to lyse strands of vitreous to cataract wounds.[4] In their series, vision improved by variable degrees in all 14 patients reported. The presence of CME was judged clinically, however, and results of pre- and postlaser fluorescein angiography were not reported for 13 of the eyes.

Because of the unpredictable natural history of aphakic CME, with erratic response to anti-inflammatory agents and frequent spontaneous improvement,[5, 6] small uncontrolled series cannot unequivocally prove the efficacy of a given technique. However, the authors' initial experience and that of their colleagues at the Massachusetts Eye and Ear Infirmary has confirmed a high rate of visual improvement after anterior segment vitreolysis. The conditions of 12 of 14 patients improved both objectively and according to the patient's own perception (Fig. 10–1). Each patient had aphakic or pseudophakic CME documented by fluorescein angiography before treatment. The interval between cataract extraction and vitreolysis ranged from 1 to 57 months. The onset of visual loss occurred within three months after cataract surgery in all cases.

The eye of the patient with the longest duration of edema, over four years, is shown before treatment in Figure 10–2. Two separate strands of vitreous were responsible for the pupillary distortion. After vitreolysis, vision improved from finger counting to 20/50, despite the long-term edema.

The interval from laser vitreolysis to visual improvement averaged nine weeks. Many patients reported dramatic improvement in vision to a stable higher level over a period of days to several weeks.

In the authors' series postlaser fluorescein angiograms were obtained for 7 of the 14 patients. Generally, macular edema resolved in those patients who

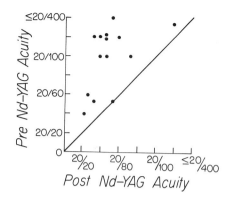

FIGURE 10–1

Scattergram of visual acuity before and after Nd-YAG laser lysis of vitreous strands to the wound for 14 aphakic and pseudophakic patients with cystoid macular edema documented by fluorescein angiography. There was no loss of vision. Twelve patients experienced an improvement in vision after treatment.

experienced nearly full recovery of vision (20/30 or better). In patients with partial recovery of vision, CME generally persisted but to a lesser degree. Table 10–1 summarizes these results.

Figure 10–3 illustrates the case of a 65-year-old aphakic patient who developed ciliary flush and contact lens intolerance with loss of vision approximately three months after intracapsular cataract extraction. He was first seen eight months after surgery, at which time an updrawn pupil and a sheet of vitreous material connected to a 150-degree cataract wound were noted (Fig. 10–3A), with a mild cellular reaction in the anterior chamber. CME with leakage into the media was documented on fluorescein angiography (Fig. 10–3B). Vision was 20/60. An Nd-YAG laser vitreolysis at 4 mJ succeeded in cutting all visible vitreous traction in two treatment sessions, and the pupil became round (Fig. 10–3C). Administration of dexamethasone 0.1 per cent drops four times daily was begun. After one week, vision varied between 20/40 and 20/60, and no further improvement occurred after eight more weeks. Repeat angiography showed persistent but reduced CME, with less leakage into the media (Fig. 10–3D). Administration of indomethacin 50 mg orally three times a day was begun, and vision improved to 20/25 within one week. The topical steroid and oral indomethacin therapy was tapered off over four weeks. Vision remained stable at 20/25, and fluorescein angiography revealed no residual CME (Fig. 10–3E).

In contrast to this case is that of a 68-year-old woman who had an uneventful intracapsular cataract extraction with an anterior chamber intraocu-

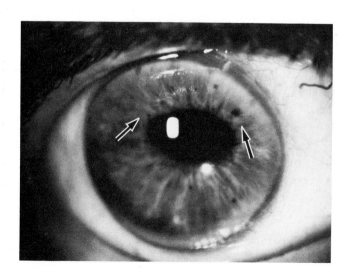

FIGURE 10–2

Pupillary distortion caused by two separate strands of vitreous to the wound (arrows). The pupil became round after treatment. Despite cystoid macular edema of 57 months' duration, vision improved from count fingers level to 20/50.

TABLE 10–1. FOURTEEN CASES OF VITREOLYSIS FOR CME

Interval from cataract surgery to CME	0–3 months
Interval from cataract surgery to laser vitreolysis	1–57 months
Interval from laser vitreolysis to stable visual improvement	
Range	2–26 weeks*
Average	9 weeks
Mode	8 weeks
Fluorescein angiographic change (7 patients evaluated)	
Resolved CME	3 patients
Reduced CME	3 patients
Unchanged	1 patient
Two treatment sessions required	5 patients

*Patient lost to follow-up between fourth and 26th week after vitreolysis.

lar lens (IOL) (Fig. 10–4). One week postoperatively an eccentric pupil was found to have developed, and vision never improved beyond 20/100 (Fig. 10–4A). A fluorescein angiogram documented CME (Fig. 10–4B). In addition to the poor central acuity, the patient was equally troubled by glare and distortion attributable to the IOL edge exposure and to unfocused light passing around the IOL optic. On examination three months after cataract surgery, gonioscopy revealed a band of vitreous adherent to the wound, apparently at the site of a wound leak with underlying bunched up iris (Color Plate IG).

Through a gonioscopy lens the YAG laser at 8 mJ dissected the vitreous adhesion at the cataract wound. The iris fell back to expose the angle (Color Plate IH). The pupil position improved markedly (Fig. 10–4C), but a portion of the optic edge remained exposed, and the patient continued to complain of glare. Re-examination revealed dense vitreous strands adherent to the posterior iris. The pupil was dilated, and through a gonioscopy lens the Nd-YAG laser at 4 mJ was used to cut as many bands as could be seen, with care taken to keep the focal point more than 4 mm from the peripheral retina. After this second session, the pupil could move fully behind the optic, and the patient no longer experienced edge glare (Fig. 10–4D). Eight weeks after completing laser treatment, using prednisolone 1 per cent drops four times a day, acuity improved to a stable level of 20/50, which has persisted without medication. Repeat fluorescein angiography showed improvement of CME, although some leakage persisted (Fig. 10–4E).

The data are inadequate to assess the role of oral administration of indomethacin in the three cases in which it was employed when no visual improvement had occurred two to three months after vitreolysis. In two cases visual improvement occurred within two weeks after the beginning of drug therapy, and the visual improvement persisted after therapy had been discontinued. In the third case—a difficult case of vitreous strands in and around an anterior chamber lens after extracapsular cataract extraction with capsule rupture and vitreous loss—vision improved from 20/100 before and after vitreolysis of 20/60 with the use of indomethacin but fell to 20/80 when use of the drug was discontinued after three months.

TECHNIQUE FOR ANTERIOR VITREOLYSIS

Preoperative Assessment. Because of the high success rate of Nd-YAG laser anterior vitreolysis in the treatment of aphakic and pseudophakic CME, it is particularly important to examine carefully for the presence of a vitreous strand to the wound in any patient with CME. The strand is usually best seen on slit lamp examination with a narrow slit beam in a darkened room, especially if pigment deposits on the vitreous strand are visible. In some cases, careful

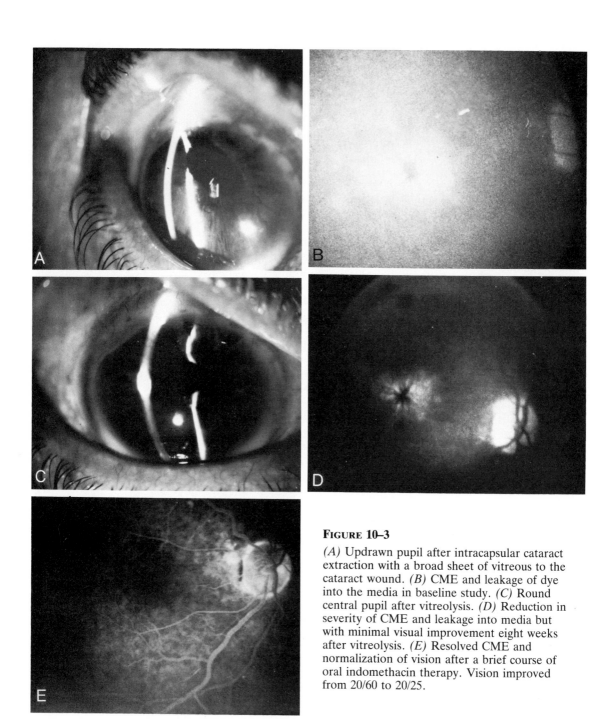

FIGURE 10–3

(A) Updrawn pupil after intracapsular cataract extraction with a broad sheet of vitreous to the cataract wound. *(B)* CME and leakage of dye into the media in baseline study. *(C)* Round central pupil after vitreolysis. *(D)* Reduction in severity of CME and leakage into media but with minimal visual improvement eight weeks after vitreolysis. *(E)* Resolved CME and normalization of vision after a brief course of oral indomethacin therapy. Vision improved from 20/60 to 20/25.

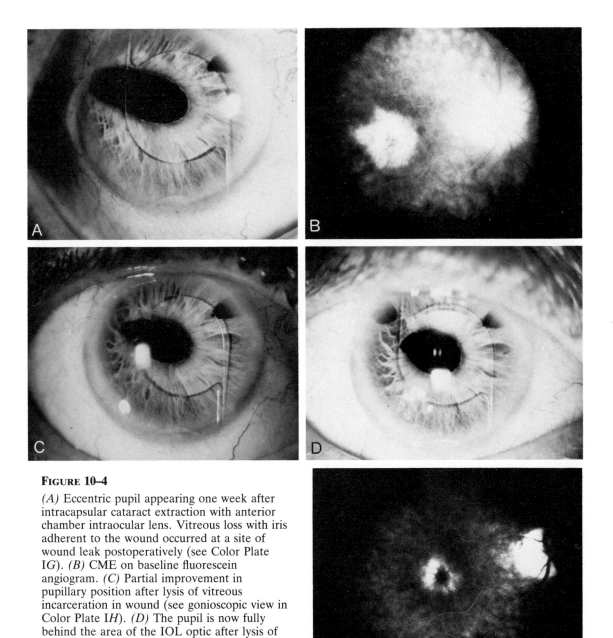

FIGURE 10–4

(A) Eccentric pupil appearing one week after intracapsular cataract extraction with anterior chamber intraocular lens. Vitreous loss with iris adherent to the wound occurred at a site of wound leak postoperatively (see Color Plate I*G*). (B) CME on baseline fluorescein angiogram. (C) Partial improvement in pupillary position after lysis of vitreous incarceration in wound (see gonioscopic view in Color Plate I*H*). (D) The pupil is now fully behind the area of the IOL optic after lysis of vitreous adhesions to the posterior iris. (E) Persistence of CME is demonstrated at a reduced level eight weeks after laser vitreolysis. Vision improved from 20/100 to 20/50.

FIGURE 10–5

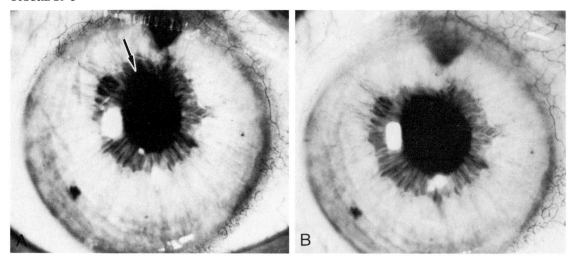

(A) A fine vitreous strand caused mild peaking of the pupil *(arrow)*. Gonioscopy showed a fine vitreous strand to the wound (Color Plate II*A*). *(B)* After laser vitreolysis, less peaking is present, but chronic change in the sphincter prevents a completely normal pupillary contour.

gonioscopy may be necessary to visualize the strand, particularly if the vitreous enters the anterior chamber through the area of a peripheral iridectomy.

Pupillary distortion may be subtle. Figure 10–5*A* shows mild peaking of a pupil, indicating a vitreous strand coming around the pupil. After vitreolysis less peaking is present, although some permanent change has occurred in the sphincter to prevent complete rounding of the pupil (Fig. 10–5*B*). (The vitreous strand responsible for this peaking of the pupil is seen in Color Plate II*A*).

Permanent changes in the iris stroma are frequent in long-term cases. Figure 10–6 shows the decreased but persistent oval shape of the pupil after

FIGURE 10–6

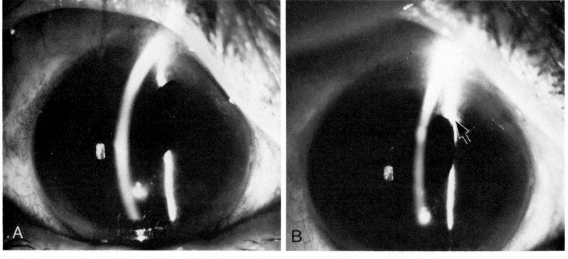

(A) An eccentric pupil caused by a vitreous strand. *(B)* After vitreolysis, depigmentation of the underlying iris stroma, present before the laser treatment, is more readily seen *(arrow)*, and the pupil remains partially distorted.

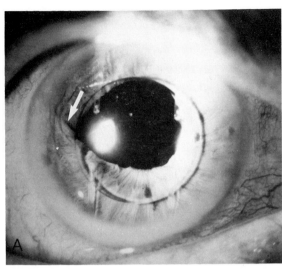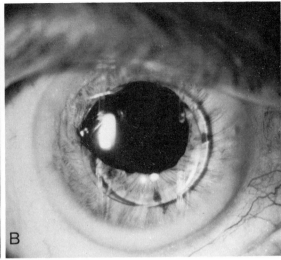

(A) The vitreous band lies flat across the iris, with vitreous tension lines emanating from the opposite side of the eye. Instead of peaking, the iris creased *(arrow)* and was held posterior to the normal iris plane in the region above the crease. *(B)* After vitreolysis, the pupillary position is unchanged, but the crease and depression are no longer present.

lysis of a vitreous strand. The iris stroma is partially depigmented locally, perhaps indicating chafing of the iris by the vitreous.

The vitreous band may distort the pupil in different ways, depending on the angle and direction of the vitreous tension. Figure 10–2 shows a "hammock" effect by two separate strands. In Figure 10–7 the vitreous causes a creasing and a shallow depression in the iris contour, which is relieved after laser treatment, although the pupil remains somewhat eccentric.

Visualization of a vitreous strand in the office is often superior to that at the laser with its extra optical components. Careful notations and sketches on strands that are difficult to visualize are helpful at the time of treatment.

Preparation of the Patient. The procedure should be explained beforehand and informed consent obtained. The patient should be told that the procedure often requires more than one session.

When the vitreous strand or band passes through the pupil, treatment is often facilitated by administration of pilocarpine 2 per cent every 15 minutes beginning two hours preoperatively. Inducing stretch of the vitreous through miosis facilitates identification of the strand and the cutting action of the laser and shows the release of the tension more definitively. In a few cases, such as that illustrated in Figure 10–4, dilation is helpful in visualizing an anterior vitreous strand in the posterior chamber.

Procedure. Figure 10–8 illustrates the three most common configurations of vitreous to the wound: (1) a small discrete strand (see Fig. 10–5 and Color Plates II*A* and *B*), (2) a broad band (see Fig. 10–3), and (3) a band with either adhesions to iris or iris entrapment behind the band (see Fig. 10–4 and Color Plates I*G* and *H*).

The laser can be directed at a vitreous strand in four general areas, shown in the inset in Figure 10–8*A*. The most reliable landmark during vitreolysis is the cataract wound, since the vitreous band or strand has to terminate at that line. The cataract wound is visualized with a gonioscopy lens (inset, Fig. 10–8*A*, pathway 1), and the laser can be fired at the wound area with a reasonable chance of successful vitreolysis. Because of the contact lens and mirror optics, the energy settings of a Q-switched Nd-YAG laser are usually 6 to 12 mJ in

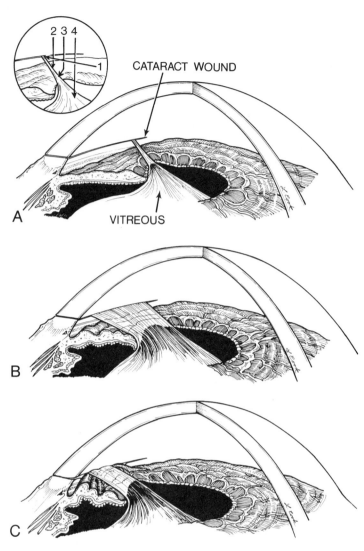

FIGURE 10–8

(A) A narrow vitreous strand to a cataract wound. The inset shows possible laser pathways for vitreolysis: (1) a gonioscopic approach, directed at the cataract wound—the location at which the vitreous strand is often the most discrete; (2) a direct approach near the limbus; (3) a direct approach in the region of the collarette; and (4) a direct approach at the pupil. This approach is rarely successful. *(B)* A broad vitreous band at the wound. *(C)* Iris pulled upward in a tentlike configuration and entrapped by the vitreous incarceration in the wound.

order to obtain adequate cutting power. The disadvantages of this technique are the requirement for use of a gonioscopy lens, which involves some extra manipulation and positioning requirements, and the subsequent commitment to use a contact lens for the completion of the treatment session, even if a different approach is needed later in the session, because of the application of gonioscopy fluid to the cornea.

If the cornea is clear near the limbus and the vitreous strand can be visualized with some clearance from the iris stroma, direct cutting without a contact lens or with a peripheral button Abraham lens may be successful along pathway 2 (inset, Fig. 10–8A). Usually 4 to 8 mJ is required. In the course of hundreds of shots along this pathway, considerable pigment may be liberated from the underlying iris stroma that will ultimately obscure the surgeon's view. Misfocused shots can cause local damage to the underlying iris or overlying cornea.

Occasionally the use of pathway 3, directed at the vitreous passing over the iris collarette, can be helpful. This is particularly true when the vitreous has formed adhesions to the collarette, pulling it forward in a tentlike formation. The close proximity of vitreous and iris make damage to the underlying iris stroma likely, but this may be clinically tolerable.

The use of pathway 4, directed at the vitreous as it passes around the pupil, is tempting but rarely successful. The vitreous traction components are poorly defined as they come around the pupil. The shock wave is ineffective at rupturing vitreous strands except directly at the laser focal point. Firing the laser immediately adjacent to the pupillary border inevitably causes low-grade capillary hemorrhage as well as release of pigment, obscuring further visualization of the area.

Successful treatment releases the tension and converts a discrete strand or band to an amorphous gelatinous appearance. Observation of the change in any iris deformation is the best indicator of successful release of tension. Hundreds of shots may be necessary to cut a large band.

Postoperative Care. Strong topical steroids (prednisolone 1 per cent, dexamethasone 0.1 per cent) are given four times daily until visual improvement occurs typically in two to three months.

Pressure rise following vitreolysis has not been well documented. In the authors' experience no patient has been observed to have a pressure increase in excess of 10 mm Hg. A drop of timolol 0.5 per cent at the time of treatment probably provides adequate prophylaxis, if desired.

The authors consider systemic administration of indomethacin 25 to 50 mg two or three times daily with meals if no visual improvement has occurred in three months and no residual vitreous traction is present. If the patient cannot tolerate indomethacin, other nonsteroidal anti-inflammatory medications can be substituted. A four-week trial of systemic medication should be adequate to assess the potential for improvement.

"Prophylactic" Vitreolysis. With the availability of laser vitreolysis, the issue has arisen of treating vitreous strands to the wound in the absence of CME, in an effort to prevent the later development of CME. Only a large long-term randomized treatment trial can scientifically determine the usefulness of such an approach. The authors consider a conservative approach to be appropriate at the present time. Many patients have been observed with vitreous strands to the wound who never develop CME. Furthermore, some patients with CME have been observed after laser vitreolysis to drop one or two lines of vision briefly after the treatment. This finding raises the question of whether the laser manipulation of the anterior vitreous has an irritative effect on the macula, with at least transient worsening of the maculopathy.

In cases of vitreous to the wound but with good vision, a baseline fluorescein angiogram is therefore recommended to document macular status. The patient's condition should then be observed closely. If visual loss develops in conjunction with new or worsened CME, laser vitreolysis can be performed promptly.

REFERENCES

1. Irvine SR. A newly defined vitreous syndrome following cataract surgery. Am J Ophthalmol 36:599–619, 1953.
2. Gass JDM, Norton EWD. Cystoid macular edema and papilledema following cataract extraction. Arch Ophthalmol 76:646–61, 1966.
3. Iliff CE. Treatment of vitreous-tug syndrome. Am J Ophthalmol 62:856–9, 1966.
4. Katzen LE, Fleischman JA, Trokel S. YAG laser treatment of cystoid macular edema. Am J Ophthalmol 95:589–92, 1983.
5. Gass JDM, Norton EWD. Follow-up study of cystoid macular edema following cataract extraction. Trans Am Acad Ophthalmol Otolaryngol 73:665–82, 1969.
6. Jacobson DR, Dellaporta A. Natural history of cystoid macular edema after cataract extraction. Am J Ophthalmol 77:445–7, 1974.

11

POSTOPERATIVE ANTERIOR CAPSULAR FRAGMENTATION AND PREOPERATIVE ANTERIOR CAPSULOTOMY

POSTOPERATIVE ANTERIOR CAPSULAR FRAGMENTATION

Retained anterior capsule after extracapsular cataract extraction can become visually significant in several ways. Capsular tags usually retract if they are small. Larger tags may continue to remain in the visual axis and be visually troublesome to the patient. These fragments can be readily severed by the Nd-YAG laser.

A dramatic case of a visually disturbing anterior capsule is illustrated in Figure 11–1. A large amount of anterior capsule was retained but not recognized at surgery. The capsule settled over the posterior chamber intraocular lens (PC IOL) optic, and because of the anterior capsular lens epithelium, rapid opacification occurred. The laser readily dissected the capsule from the IOL optic; the capsule showed no adhesion to the polymethylmethacrylate (PMMA). Despite multiple shots at the surface, no IOL damage was observed. The anterior propagation of plasma (see Chapter 3) explains the lack of IOL damage associated with work on its anterior surface (see also Fig. 9–10). Rather than cut a large fragment free in the anterior chamber, the capsule was left attached at one corner. By placing shots in the anterior chamber the pressure wave was utilized to cause the capsule to curl up upon itself and subsequently adhere in that position.

A fragment of capsule can also traumatize the corneal endothelium with resultant edema, as shown in Color Plate IIC. The Nd-YAG laser at 3 mJ readily cut the capsular fragment, and the edema resolved. A tag of capsule remained adherent to the endothelium (Color Plate IID).

TECHNIQUE FOR ANTERIOR CAPSULAR FRAGMENTATION

Preparation of the Patient. The procedure should be explained and informed consent obtained. No special preparation is routinely required.

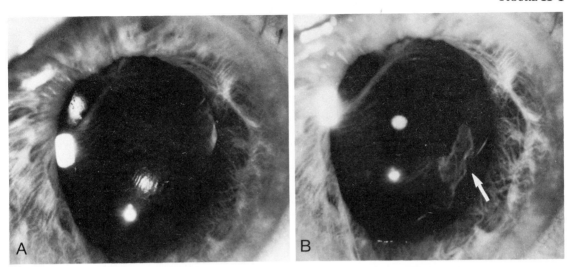

(A) A large remnant of retained anterior capsule has opacified over the anterior surface of a posterior chamber IOL optic. (B) The central capsule was cut free by sequential 3 mJ shots beginning in the upper left corner and progressing to the lower right. The capsule was left uncut at the lower right corner. Pulses in the anterior chamber were used to cause the capsule to curl up over itself (arrow).

Technique. The anterior capsule fragments generally are disrupted with 1 to 4 mJ in only a few pulses. A gonioscopy lens is occasionally useful to properly direct the laser beam to the target.

Postoperative Care. Inflammatory reaction and pressure rise are usually minimal and should be treated as they occur.

PREOPERATIVE ANTERIOR CAPSULOTOMY

Aron-Rosa was the first to report using the Nd-YAG laser for anterior capsulotomy before extracapsular cataract extraction.[1] Preoperative anterior capsulotomy was said to facilitate extracapsular surgery by softening the cortex and reducing surgical time. The potential for a reduced rate of postoperative posterior capsule opacification was suggested by an incidence of 7 per cent opacification in a follow-up period of six months to two years.

Aron-Rosa's procedure was to employ 100 to 200 shots to form a continuous opening in the capsule 1 to 24 hours before surgery. She used the laser to partially fragment a hard nucleus at the time of the anterior capsulotomy. Patients were reportedly pretreated with indomethacin 500 mg daily for six weeks preoperatively. (This dose greatly exceeds the drug manufacturer's recommendations. The basis for a long period of pretreatment at a high dose is unclear and this practice may be hazardous.) In a series of 200 patients, Aron-Rosa found no changes in endothelial cell counts, but data were not given. Intraocular pressure was found to have increased in 20 patients with intumescent cataracts when the opening was made 24 hours before surgery but not in 15 patients with capsulotomy performed two hours before surgery. No pressure change was noted in 105 patients with immature nuclear, cortical, and subcapsular cataracts. The postoperative course was unremarkable in all cases.

The original recommendation by Aron-Rosa was that advanced cataracts with cortical liquefaction have preoperative laser anterior capsulotomy less than three hours before surgery; anterior capsulotomy in immature cataracts could be performed hours to a day before surgery.

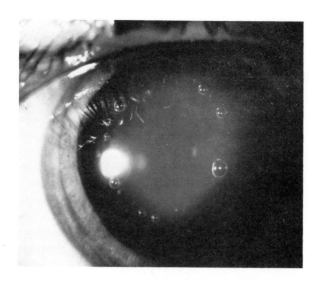

FIGURE 11–2

Appearance of lens immediately after Nd-YAG laser anterior capsulotomy in a patient with subluxated lenses and Weill-Marchesani syndrome. Note the eccentric location of the laser marks relative to the pupil as a result of the subluxation of the lens. (Courtesy of Paul M. Woodward.)

Laser anterior capsulotomy in advance of cataract surgery to cause rapid cortical softening is somewhat analogous to the old procedure of "needling" a cataract days to weeks before extracapsular cataract extraction. In that era, irrigation-aspiration instruments and operative microscopic visualization were not available, and the "needling" procedure was abandoned once successful intracapsular cataract extraction was developed. Extracapsular surgery only regained popularity when irrigation-aspiration techniques allowed thorough removal of immature cortex.

Aron-Rosa now rarely employs preoperative laser anterior capsulotomy.* She developed the technique at a time when simple irrigation was used to remove the cortex. Since that time she has adopted modern irrigation-aspiration techniques. She found that preoperative anterior capsulotomy caused the cortex to acquire a gummy consistency, which made irrigation-aspiration more difficult. Overall, Aron-Rosa now prefers operative anterior capsulotomy, nucleus expression, and irrigation-aspiration cortical stripping over preoperative laser anterior capsulotomy, nucleus expression, and simple irrigation of the softened cortex.

The Q-switched or mode-locked Nd-YAG lasers currently employed cannot substantially fragment or soften a senile nucleus. Expression or sonication of the nucleus must still be employed.

Several American ophthalmologists have adopted and modified preoperative laser anterior capsulotomy. Paul Woodward and Robert Drews routinely

*D Aron-Rosa 1984: personal communication.

TABLE 11–1. INDICATIONS AND CONTRAINDICATIONS FOR PREOPERATIVE LASER ANTERIOR CAPSULOTOMY

Indications
1. Hydration of the cortex in immature cataracts
2. Anterior capsulotomy without zonule damage in cataracts with weak zonules or subluxation

Contraindications
1. Mature or hypermature cataracts
2. Preoperative glaucoma
3. History of intraocular inflammation
4. Poor pupillary dilation
5. Lack of medical and anesthesia clearance for cataract surgery before performing laser anterior capsulotomy
6. Medical, physical, or emotional factors that may cause cancellation of the cataract surgery after capsulotomy has been performed

TABLE 11–2. PROPOSED ADVANTAGES OF PREOPERATIVE LASER ANTERIOR CAPSULOTOMY

1. The location and extent of anterior capsular opening are precise.
2. There is no stress on zonules.
3. Cortical hydration facilitates cortical removal by irrigation techniques.
4. Nucleus expression may be eased.
5. Posterior capsule clarity may be improved, and postoperative capsule opacification may be reduced or delayed.

open the anterior capsule hours to days before cataract extraction. Color Plates II*E* and *F* illustrate cortical hydration 24 hours after laser anterior capsulotomy. This is in distinction to a laser anterior capsulotomy performed immediately before the patient enters the operating room—a variation in technique that allows a precise capsular opening but does not allow time for physical changes in the cortex.

In addition to use of laser anterior capsulotomy in routine cataract surgery, Woodward has reported a specific indication.[2] A 28-year-old man with Weill-Marchesani syndrome and subluxated lenses required cataract extraction. In the presence of weak and absent zonules, conventional bent needle or scissor anterior capsulotomy often results in further loss of zonules with the potential of vitreous loss and possible full dislocation of the lens. Vitreous loss is also common in intracapsular extraction of subluxated lenses, particularly in young patients. After using his own laser anterior capsulotomy technique, Woodward was able to successfully perform the remainder of the extracapsular cataract extraction with an intact posterior capsule, avoiding vitreous loss. Figure 11–2 shows the immediate appearance of the subluxated lens after the laser treatment.

Table 11–1 gives the current indications and contraindications for laser anterior capsulotomy in advance of extracapsular cataract extraction. Table 11–2 itemizes advantages claimed for this technique, and Table 11–3 lists the complications. In addition to the potential hazards of high intraocular pressure, inflammation, a small pupil at the time of surgery, and possible trauma to the corneal endothelium, unforeseen problems may prevent completion of operation as scheduled, leading to phacolytic glaucoma or phacoanaphylaxis. Examples of such problems include complications of anesthesia, including retrobulbar hemorrhage after injection, unforeseen medical complications such as myocardial infarction, and emotional or behavioral disturbance in the patient that leads to refusal or inability to complete the surgery.

The authors have no personal experience with preoperative laser anterior capsulotomy. Paul M. Woodward, M.D., has shared his typical preoperative protocol and laser and surgical technique:

TECHNIQUE FOR PREOPERATIVE ANTERIOR CAPSULOTOMY

Preparation of the Patient. Indomethacin 75 mg orally and timolol 0.5 per cent topically are given 90 minutes before laser treatment. Phenylephrine 2.5 per cent and cyclopentolate 1 per cent are administered every 15 minutes until the pupil is fully dilated.

TABLE 11–3. COMPLICATIONS OF PREOPERATIVE LASER ANTERIOR CAPSULOTOMY

1. Intraocular pressure elevation at the time of surgery
2. Intraocular inflammation and pain
3. Miosis interfering with extracapsular surgery
4. Phacolytic glaucoma or phacoanaphylaxis if surgery is not completed as scheduled
5. Possible corneal endothelial injury with peripheral shots in shallow anterior chamber

TABLE 11–4. LASER ANTERIOR CAPSULOTOMY AND CATARACT EXTRACTION:
TYPICAL PREPARATION AND TECHNIQUES*

Preparation for anterior capsulotomy
1. Administration of indomethacin 75 mg orally and timolol 0.5% topically 90 minutes before laser treatment.
2. Administration of phenylephrine 2.5% and cyclopentolate 1% topically every 15 minutes until dilation.

Laser anterior capsulotomy
1. Laser is set for minimal energy necessary to form vacuoles and rupture the anterior capsule (1–3 mJ).
2. If cortex is clear, the laser is focused at areas posterior to the anterior capsule, and central vacuoles are formed.
3. Anterior capsulotomy is made by 100 to 200 interconnecting shots no closer than 2 mm to the pupil margin.
4. The procedure is usually performed 24 hours preoperatively. For intumescent cataracts, laser capsulotomy is performed only two hours preoperatively. Hypermature cataracts are not treated with laser anterior capsulotomy.

Therapy between anterior capsulotomy and cataract extraction
1. Intraocular pressure is measured two hours after laser treatment. Pressure rise is treated as indicated with acetazolamide and timolol.
2. Cycloplegics and mydriatics are used as needed to maintain large pupil size.

Special elements in cataract surgical technique
1. Large wound.
2. Irrigation with 23-gauge smooth olive tip cannula and gravity infusion of balanced salt irrigant.
3. Aspiration if needed with a 0.2-mm port cannula.

*Courtesy of Paul M. Woodward.

Procedure. Laser anterior capsulotomy is usually performed the day before cataract extraction. The laser is directed coaxially and focused on the anterior capsule in a position at least 2 mm central to the margin of the pupil. The lowest energy setting that ruptures the capsule is then used. As many as 100 to 200 shots are rapidly placed to create an interconnecting series of capsulotomies. If the cortex is clear, the laser is initially focused posterior to the anterior capsule and fired to create vacuoles under the capsule, as shown in Color Plate II*E*. The capsulotomy is then performed. If the cortex is opaque, the capsulotomy alone is performed.

Hypermature cataracts and patients with glaucoma are not treated by laser anterior capsulotomy. Laser capsulotomy is used for intumescent cataracts no more than two hours before surgery.

Therapy Between Laser Anterior Capsulotomy and Cataract Extraction. Intraocular pressure is measured two hours after the anterior capsulotomy. Acetazolamide and timolol are administered as indicated if a pressure rise occurs. Cycloplegics are given as required by the inflammatory response to maintain large pupil size. The surgeon must be prepared to perform emergency cataract surgery for intractable elevation of intraocular pressure or severe inflammation.

Special Elements in Cataract Surgical Technique. A large wound is needed to irrigate the cortex. Irrigation is performed by a 23-gauge smooth blunt-tipped cannula with gravity infusion of a balanced salt irrigant. In most cases, aspiration is unnecessary. If aspiration is necessary to strip residual cortex, a small tip such as a 0.2-mm port McIntyre cannula is used because gummy hydrated cortex does not occlude larger ports well.

Table 11–4 summarizes the elements of patient preparation and laser and surgical technique.

REFERENCES
1. Aron-Rosa D. Use of a pulsed neodymium-YAG laser for anterior capsulotomy before extracapsular cataract extraction. J Am Intraocul Implant Soc 7:332–3, 1981.
2. Woodward P. Nd-YAG laser anterior capsulotomy in Marchesani syndrome. J Am Intraocul Implant Soc 10:215–7, 1984.

12

OTHER ANTERIOR SEGMENT APPLICATIONS

CUTTING IOL HAPTICS

Removal of an anterior chamber intraocular lens (IOL) may require cutting the haptic if the IOL feet have fibrosed into the angle, which is often the case when postoperative pathology necessitates IOL removal. The Nd-YAG laser may facilitate removal by cutting the haptics located farthest from the surgical opening.

Figure 12–1 illustrates a case of fibrovascular ingrowth from a wound. The ingrowth began two months after successful treatment of endophthalmitis after intracapsular cataract extraction and anterior chamber IOL implantation. The fibrous tissue rapidly covered the IOL and encased the haptic feet above and below with a fibrovascular membrane in the angle. To avoid the difficulty of reaching across the anterior chamber with strong scissors to cut the inferior haptics or the necessity of creating a second wound below, the laser was used to sever the extruded polymethylmethacrylate haptics as close as possible to the limbus at the 5 and 7 o'clock positions. The patient subsequently was taken to the operating room. There a superior wound allowed straightforward cutting of the superior haptics with scissors and removal of the IOL.

Cutting of polymethylmethacrylate or polypropylene haptics usually requires 6 to 12 mJ and 25 to 100 shots. The haptics often appear to be thinning and focally vaporizing, as well as cracking from the pressure wave.

If the surgeon anticipates that the haptic material is sufficiently flexible that it can uncurl and slide out of the tissue in the angle that encases it, then only one arm of the inferior haptic need be cut. At surgery, once the superior haptics are cut, the IOL can be rotated by a hook to slide the entire haptic out of the angle. In this manner, no haptic material is left in the eye.

IOL REPOSITIONING

The pressure wave generated by the Nd-YAG laser pulse can manipulate the position of intraocular structures. This ability proved useful in a case of iris capture of a posterior chamber IOL. The iris capture shown in Figure 12–2A occurred after dilation for routine posterior capsulotomy. The pupil could not

FIGURE 12–1

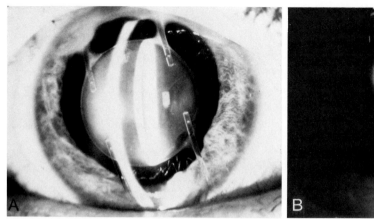
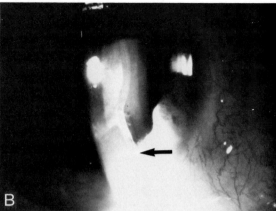

(A) Fibrous tissue from the superior wound has grown across this anterior chamber IOL
to encase the haptic inserts in the angle. *(B)* The Nd-YAG laser cut the inferior haptic
inserts near the limbus preoperatively *(arrow).* At subsequent surgery a superior wound
was used to approach and cut the superior haptic inserts and to remove the lens.

be redilated beyond the edge of the optic. Patient positioning and oral
administration of hyperosmotic agents had no effect. Manipulation with a
cotton swab over the ciliary sulcus failed to identify a haptic pressure point
that would cause the IOL to move. The patient was taken back to the Nd-
YAG laser, which was aimed at an area oriented approximately 1 mm centrally
from the edge of the optic, just anterior to the IOL surface. After a single
poorly focused shot had been unsuccessful, another single 6-mJ shot retropulsed
the optic behind the iris, which reacted with miosis, trapping the optic in its
proper position in the posterior chamber.

REOPENING FAILED FILTERS

Directed through a gonioscopy lens, an Nd-YAG laser may be able to
reopen a blocked filtering sclerostomy site. Cohn and Aron-Rosa first reported

FIGURE 12–2

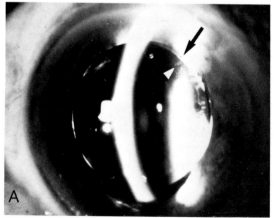
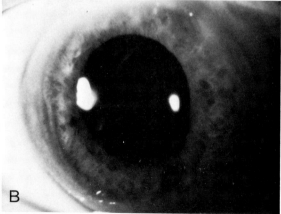

(A) Iris capture of the optic of a posterior chamber IOL *(arrow).* A single 6-mJ pulse
focused at an area just anterior to the lens surface, approximately 1 mm centrally from
the optic edge *(arrowhead),* retropulsed the optic behind the iris. *(B)* The IOL is now in
proper position behind the iris.

successful restoration of filtration when the sclerostomy itself was visibly occluded by a membrane.[1] Praeger subsequently reported using 300 to 500 shots from a mode-locked Nd-YAG laser to restore filtration in four patients who were losing their filtering blebs with increasing intraocular pressure within six weeks of surgery.[2] One of these was a case of vitreous material plugging a sclerostomy site; the other three cases involved membranes in the anterior chamber that occluded the sclerostomy and were visible on gonioscopy.

Glaucoma filters most often fail owing to membranous proliferation of the episclera across the sclerostomy site.[3, 4] The Nd-YAG laser would not be expected to be able to restore filtration in these cases.

Application of the Nd-YAG laser to failing filters may cause bleeding and inflammation with the risk of increased intraocular pressure and further failure of the filter. A 9-year-old boy with unilateral congenital ectropion uveae associated with glaucoma had undergone successful posterior lip sclerectomy after three goniotomies failed to normalize the intraocular pressure. After several years, however, the bleb began to flatten, and intraocular pressure rose to 26 mm Hg. Digital pressure transiently lowered the pressure to 22 mm Hg. Figure 12–3A shows the initial appearance of the low bleb. Gonioscopy revealed a slender tongue of pigmented tissue extending from the peripheral iridectomy to the sclerostomy site, which appeared occluded. Nine shots at 6 mJ and nine shots at 11 mJ appeared to open the sclerostomy internally. Upon removal of the gonioscopy lens a large diffuse filtering bleb was found. Intraocular pressure had fallen to 12 mm Hg. Within several minutes a small strand of clotted blood was found to have extended from the sclerostomy site across the anterior chamber down to the inferior angle (Fig. 12–3B), and a small subconjunctival hemorrhage could be seen under the bleb (Fig. 12–3C). One half hour after

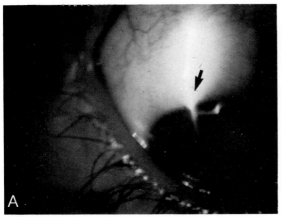

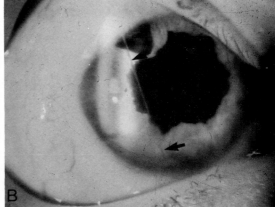

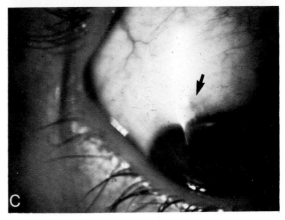

FIGURE 12–3

(A) Appearance of filtering bleb before laser treatment (arrow) in a patient with congenital ectropion uveae. (B) A clot extends across the anterior chamber from the sclerostomy site after Nd-YAG laser treatment of the occluded opening (arrows). (C) The appearance of the filtering bleb after laser treatment shows subconjunctival hemorrhage (arrow).

the treatment the bleb was found once again to be flat, and the intraocular pressure had risen to 47 mm Hg. Additional mediation reduced the pressure to its pre–laser-treatment level. In follow-up the filter continued to function, however, and intraocular pressure averaged 16 mm Hg two months after the laser procedure.

Experience with this procedure is too preliminary to use as a basis for generalization about the frequency with which this approach will be indicated, the long-term success rate, or complications. In selected cases this technique may forestall the necessity for further surgery to treat glaucoma. It should be restricted, however, to cases that are so severe that reoperation with conventional surgery is the only alternative, and to the unusual cases in which internal blockage of the sclerostomy is the basis for failure of the filter.

STAGED FILTERING SCLEROTOMY

Weber and coworkers have reported a two-staged glaucoma filtering technique that offers a reduced incidence of shallow or flat chamber in their hands. At surgery the sclerotomy is made with only partial thickness, leaving a very thin walled residual barrier between the anterior chamber and the subconjunctival space. The day after surgery, the Nd-YAG laser directed through a gonioscopy lens is fired at the sclerotomy site to complete the operation and establish a filtering sclerostomy into the subconjunctival space.

The rationale for this procedure is that the day between the two stages allows the conjunctival wound to seal itself, reducing the frequency of excess filtration and subsequent loss of the chamber. This group uses a fornix-based conjunctival flap, rather than the more common limbus-based conjunctival flap. In the case of a fornix-based flap, it might particularly be expected that the healing period before filtration begins would reduce bleb leaks and the rate of formation of shallow chambers.

TRABECULOPUNCTURE, CYCLODIALYSIS, AND GONIOTOMY

In open angle glaucoma, the Q-switched ruby laser of Krasnov and later the Q-switched Nd-YAG laser of Fankhauser and coworkers have been able to achieve puncture from the anterior chamber into Schlemm's canal.[6–9] Intraocular pressure rapidly falls to low normal levels when such "trabeculopuncture" is achieved. The uniform experience to date has been that pressure returns to pretreatment levels several months after the laser trabeculopuncture. This return is associated with a visible filling-in of the trabeculopuncture site. No treatment protocol has yet been successful in arresting this healing response. Histopathologic studies of monkeys show closure of the trabeculopuncture sites by endothelial cell proliferation.[9]

Fankhauser also has attempted to perform cyclodialysis with the Nd-YAG laser.[9, 10] Using multimode Q-switched pulses between 40 to 60 mJ, he caused localized detachment of the ciliary body with formation of a cleft in the suprachoroidal space. However, a sustained decrease in intraocular pressure occurred in only one of 31 eyes treated; in the other 30 cases, the pressure rose after treatment. This procedure was therefore abandoned. Fellman, Starita, and Spaeth reported a case in which the Nd-YAG laser was apparently successful in reopening a failed cyclodialysis cleft after trabeculoplasty by Watson's technique.[11]

In principle the short-pulsed Nd-YAG laser may be capable of cutting Barkan's membrane in cases of congenital glaucoma. However, the laser is not usually situated in a suitable location for general anesthesia, and corneal edema may limit the visualization and focusing necessary to achieve optical breakdown. Cases of juvenile glaucoma with an abnormal membrane in the angle may also be candidates for Nd-YAG laser goniotomy. Clinical use of laser goniotomy has not been reported to date but remains an interesting theoretical application.

REFERENCES

1. Cohn HC, Aron-Rosa D. Reopening blocked trabeculectomy sites with the YAG laser. Am J Ophthalmol 95:293–4, 1983.
2. Praeger DL. The opening of closed filtering blebs using the neodymium-YAG laser. Ophthalmology 91:373–7, 1984.
3. Maumenee AE. External filtering operations for glaucoma: The mechanism of function and failure. Trans Am Ophthalmol Soc 58:319–25, 1960.
4. Flaxel JT, Swan KC. Limbal wound healing after cataract extraction: A histologic study. Arch Ophthalmol 81:653–9, 1969.
5. Weber PA, Keates RH, Opremcek EM, Kapetansky FM, Szymanski C. Two-stage neodymium-YAG laser trabeculotomy. Ophthalmic Surg 14:591–4, 1983.
6. Krasnov M. Q-switched laser goniopuncture. Arch Ophthalmol 92:37–41, 1974.
7. Krasnov M. Q-switched laser iridectomy and Q-switched laser goniopuncture. Adv Ophthalmol 34:192–6, 1977.
8. Fankhauser F, Roussel P, Steffen J, Van der Zypen E, Chrenkova A. Clinical studies on the efficiency of high power laser radiation upon some structures of the anterior segment of the eye. Int Ophthalmol 3:129–39, 1981.
9. Van der Zypen E, Fankhauser F. The ultrastructural features of laser trabeculopuncture and cyclodialysis. Ophthalmologica 179:189–200, 1979.
10. Fankhauser F. The Q-switched laser: Principles and clinical results. *In* Trokel SL (ed.). YAG Laser Ophthalmic Microsurgery. Norwalk, CT: Appleton-Century-Crofts, 1983, pp 101–46.
11. Fellman RL, Starita RJ, Spaeth GL. Reopening cyclodialysis cleft with Nd:YAG laser following trabeculectomy. Ophthalmic Surg 15:285–8, 1984.

13

POSTERIOR SEGMENT APPLICATIONS

The use of the short-pulsed neodymium-YAG laser to section posterior vitreous membranes presents potential risks and technical challenges greater than those encountered in the use of the laser to cut membranes in the pupillary plane or anterior vitreous. As detailed in Chapter 4, when working in the pupillary plane (that is, between 17 and 20 mm from the retinal surface), the risk of retinal injury is quite low even at high pulse energies, since the divergence of the laser light after the focal point ensures that retinal irradiance is below the threshold for damage. Microplasma formation also provides a partial reduction in the transmission of energy along the beam path in both Q-switched and mode-locked laser systems. The risk of fundus injury increases exponentially as the laser is fired at points closer to the retinal surface, since the beam has a shorter distance over which to diverge. Retinal irradiance increases as a square function as the focal point approaches the retina. Moreover, if the optical breakdown zone is too close to the surface of the retina, acoustic and shock waves can propagate into the retina and choroid to produce choroidal hemorrhage or disruption of the retina.

Indications. The goals of traditional vitreous surgery are removal of opaque vitreous humor to restore a clear optical pathway and the sectioning, delamination, or removal of membranes producing clinically significant retinal traction. For cases with proliferative vitreoretinopathy such as in diabetes, most surgeons now favor as complete a vitrectomy as possible, in which the posterior vitreous is severed from all connections with the vitreous base, and removal of the scaffold for present and future vitreous membrane proliferation.[1] However, vitrectomy is not without risks and, in principle, the concept of a noninvasive approach for treatment of some eyes with posterior vitreous membranes is an attractive one.

The Nd-YAG laser may be useful in cutting discrete vitreous membranes (without a significant vascular component) associated with clinically significant retinal traction. The number of such cases is small compared with the large number of eyes with extensive or complex posterior vitreous membranes. The authors' experimental studies[2] and clinical experience suggest that heavily vascularized membranes, such as those seen in proliferative diabetic retinopathy, should be avoided unless the vessels can be successfully obliterated by photocoagulation prior to the pulsed YAG laser treatment. However, direct treatment of intravitreal vessels with the argon laser has met with only very limited success.[3] There is little evidence to suggest that photodisruption of diffusely hemorrhagic or opaque vitreous facilitates restoration of a clear optical pathway.

TECHNIQUE OF POSTERIOR SEGMENT VITREOLYSIS

Preoperative Assessment. There are a number of technical requirements for photodisruption of posterior segment vitreous membranes. The media anterior to the target should be clear, and the pupil should be well dilated. The patient must be highly cooperative, since the treatment sessions tend to be longer in duration than for anterior segment cases.

Membranes should be discrete and avascular. Fluorescein angiography may be useful in establishing the absence of vessels in the membranes to be treated. Membranes that are under tension are easiest to cut; membranes that are freely floating or highly fibrous are the most difficult to cut.

Careful preoperative examination with the indirect ophthalmoscope and, most importantly, the fundus contact lens through which the treatment is delivered, is essential. The purpose of the examination is to formulate a therapeutic strategy, in which the points are selected at which the membranes are to be dissected and a safe working distance to both the retina and the lens is maintained.

It is difficult to develop firm guidelines for the pulse energy at a given focal point from the retina that will be entirely safe. In extensive studies with membranes in animal eyes, the authors were able to cut vitreous membranes up to 4 mm from the retinal surface with the use of single pulse energies of up to 4 mJ without fluorescein angiographic evidence of injury.[2] Fankhauser states that he has frequently noted retinal hemorrhage at distances of 3 to 4 mm from the retinal surface even when using low pulse energies.[4] The danger of retinal or choroidal hemorrhage increases rapidly (exponentially) as work is performed closer to the retinal surface.

Preparation of the Patient. The pupil is dilated with a topical cycloplegic and a mydriatic one half hour to one hour prior to treatment. Topical anesthesia only is generally employed, but retrobulbar anesthesia can be used if necessary for akinesia.

Technique. The authors prefer to peform this treatment using a contact lens with an anterior radius of curvature of 18 mm. For treatments in the periphery, a three-mirror contact lens may be employed. Use of a flat fundus contact lens should be avoided, since it decreases the angle of divergence of the beam after the focal point.

The general approach is to select a treatment point that is at a maximal distance from the surface of the retina and from the posterior surface of the lens. Working over the macula should be avoided. It is desirable to work over an area of previous photocoagulation if possible. The authors typically use single pulse energies of 3 to 6 mJ, delivered in single shots (Fig. 13–1). Use of burst mode may make cutting faster, but the adverse consequences of a misdirected burst shot are greater than for a single shot. Because posterior segment vitreous membranes tend to be complex and fibrous, hundreds or even thousands of pulse applications may be necessary to transect a membrane. Multiple treatment sessions are often necessary.

Focusing and localization are two significant challenges when cutting deep vitreous membranes. Accurate focusing of the laser is more difficult than in the anterior segment, particularly when cutting thin or highly transparent membranes or when working in the fundus periphery. If clear focus without induced astigmatism is not achieved, optical breakdown will not occur since the irradiance necessary to initiate plasma formation is not achieved. Use of a dual-

FIGURE 13–1

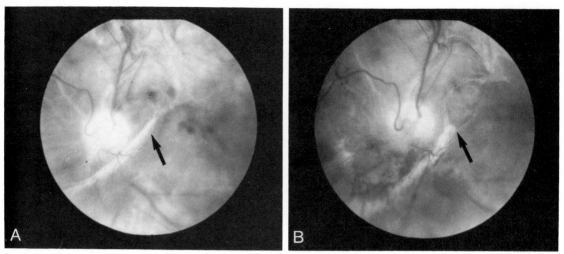

(A) This patient developed a fibrovascular strand *(arrow)* that detached the superior part of the macula after superior hemicentral vein occlusion. *(B)* Postoperative appearance after cutting of the strand with 30 Q-switched pulses of 5 mJ. Note the cut end of the strand *(arrow)* and the reduction of retinal traction. (*A, B* Courtesy of Thomas A. Hanscom.)

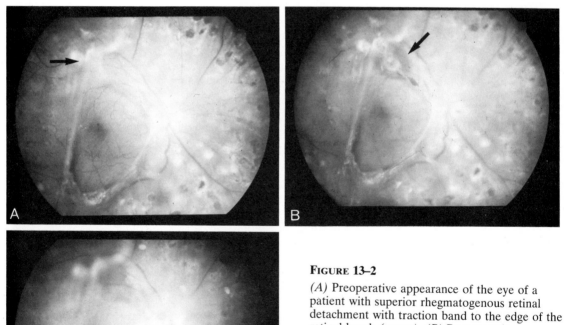

FIGURE 13–2

(A) Preoperative appearance of the eye of a patient with superior rhegmatogenous retinal detachment with traction band to the edge of the retinal break *(arrow)*. *(B)* Postoperative appearance (after one hour). Note the choroidal hemorrhage just inside the superior retinal arcade *(arrow)*. This complication occurred at a pulse energy of 5 mJ. *(C)* One month after treatment, choroidal hemorrhage had partially resolved without further complication.

beam or other multiple-beam focusing system facilitates accurate aim. Localization of the laser's focal point relative to the surface of the retina may be difficult. An optical micrometer system aided by preoperative A-scan biometry, can measure the displacement of the laser focal point from a reference point such as the retina or from the cornea or lens. This device can be quite helpful in localization, particularly if this measurement is displayed in real time in the oculars of the slit lamp.

Complications. A number of serious complications can result from YAG laser photodisruption in the posterior segment. Retinal injury can occur either when the operator is focusing correctly while cutting a membrane close to the retinal surface at a high pulse energy or when the surgeon is inadvertently focusing closer to the retina than is recommended. Choroidal and retinal hemorrhage and hole formation are the two most frequently observed complications (Fig. 13–2). These hemorrhages may be produced by the propagation of acoustic transients into the retina and choroid with vessel rupture or by the high level of irradiance. Choroidal hemorrhage has been recognized for some time as a characteristic form of suprathreshold retinal injury produced by lasers operating in the nanosecond or picosecond time domains.[5] Choroidal hemorrhage may be associated with rupture of Bruch's membrane and in human eyes carries with it the potential for subsequent chorioretinal or choriovitreal neovascularization.[6] If choroidal hemorrhage is observed to occur during treatment, it usually can be stopped by increasing the pressure that holds the contact lens to the eye.

Punctate retinal hemorrhages are often observed when membranes are cut close to the retinal surface. Delayed onset of retinal injury 24 hours following YAG laser photodisruption of deep vitreous membranes has been reported. Such retinal injury consisted of white spots at the level of the retinal pigment epithelium, which stained in the late phase of the fluorescein angiogram.[7]

Contrary to some claims, there is little evidence that mode-locked Nd-YAG lasers are safer than Q-switched lasers for work in the posterior segment. In fact, one experimental study suggested that the threshold for retinal injury was higher for mode-locked pulses when compared with Q-switched pulses of equivalent energy producing optical breakdown at the same distance from the retinal surface.[8]

In the phakic eye, injury to the lens is of concern. Focal lens injury during YAG laser surgery of posterior vitreous membranes has been reported.[9] It is desirable to keep the laser at least 4 mm beyond the posterior surface of the crystalline lens.

Postoperative Care. Following the treatment, the patient should be carefully re-examined to see whether the initial surgical goals have been achieved. Further treatment with the laser may be considered as well as a conventional vitreous surgical approach.

REFERENCES

1. Machemer R, Aaberg T. Vitrectomy. 2nd ed. New York: Grune & Stratton, 1979, p 22.
2. Puliafito CA, Wasson PJ, Steinert RF, Gragoudas ES. Nd-YAG Laser surgery on experimental vitreous membranes. Arch Ophthalmol 102:843–47, 1984.
3. Hamilton AM, Townsend C, Khoury D, Gould E. Treatment of new vessels on the disc in diabetic retinopathy. Trans Ophthal Soc UK 96:228–35, 1976.
4. Fankhauser F. The Q-switched laser: Principles and clinical results. *In* Trokel S (ed.). YAG Laser Ophthalmic Microsurgery. Norwalk, CT: Appleton-Century-Crofts, 1983, pp 128–31.
5. Gibbons WB, Allen RG. Retinal damage from suprathreshold Q-switched laser exposure. Health Phys 35:461–9, 1978.
6. Dizon-Moore RV, Jampol L, Goldberg MF. Chorioretinal and choriovitreal neovascularization. Arch Ophthalmol 99:842–79, 1981.
7. Jampol LM, Goldberg MF, Jednock N. Retinal damage from a Q-switched YAG laser. Am J Ophthalmol 96:326–9, 1983.
8. Bonner RF, Meyers SM, Gaasterland DE. Threshold for retinal damage associated with the use of high-power neodymium YAG lasers in the vitreous. Am J Ophthalmol 96:153–9, 1983.
9. Little HL, Jack RL. Q-switched Nd-YAG laser in vitreous surgery. Presented at the American Academy of Ophthalmology, Annual Meeting, November 1983.

APPENDIX

Abbreviations and Symbols
Used in the Text

AC IOL	anterior chamber intraocular lens
Ar	Argon
c	speed of light (3×10^8 cm per second in vacuum)
°C	degrees Celsius
cm	centimeter
CME	cystoid macular edema
CO_2	carbon dioxide
E	electron atomic energy level
ECCE	extracapsular cataract extraction
Er-YLF	erbium-yttrium-lanthanum-fluoride
F	fluoride
h	Planck's constant (6.6×10^{-34} joules $\cdot$ second)
He-Ne	helium-neon laser
Hg	mercury
H PD	hematoporphyrin derivative
Hz	Hertz (cycles per second)
ICCE	intracapsular cataract extraction
IOL	intraocular lens
J	joule
km	kilometer
Kr	krypton
λ	lambda (wavelength)
m	meter
mg	milligram
mJ	millijoule
mm	millimeter
mrad	milliradian
msec	millisecond
mw	milliwatt
μ	mu (micron)
ν	nu (frequency)

Nd-YAG	neodymium-yttrium-aluminum-garnet
nm	nanometer (10^{-9} m)
nsec	nanosecond (10^{-9} seconds)
PC IOL	posterior chamber intraocular lens
PMMA	polymethylmethacralate
p.r.n.	pro re nata (as the need arises)
PRT	photoradiation therapy
psec	picosecond (10^{-12} seconds)
Q	quality
sec	second
TEM	Transverse Electro-Magnetic
UV	ultraviolet
V	volt
W	watt
YAG	yttrium-aluminum-garnet

INDEX

Page numbers in *italics* indicate illustrations. Page numbers followed by t indicate tables.